The Complete Plant Based Diet Cookbook with Pictures

6 Books in 1: 300+ Delicious Recipes to Purify and Energize Your Body with Vegan and Plant Based Food

Frank Smith

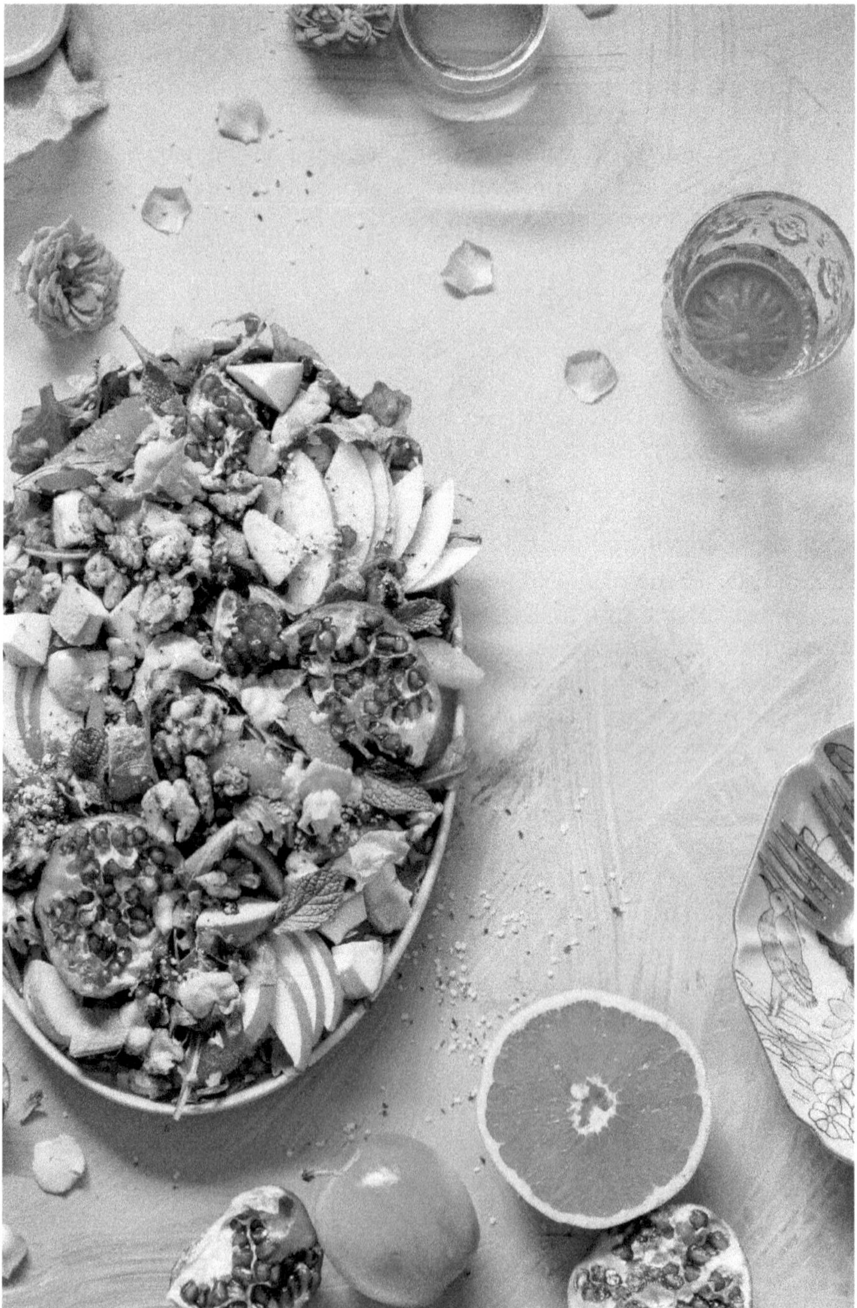

Plant Based Diet Cookbook for Beginners with Pictures

Tasty and Quick Recipes to Purify and Energize Your Body

Frank Smith

Table Of Contents

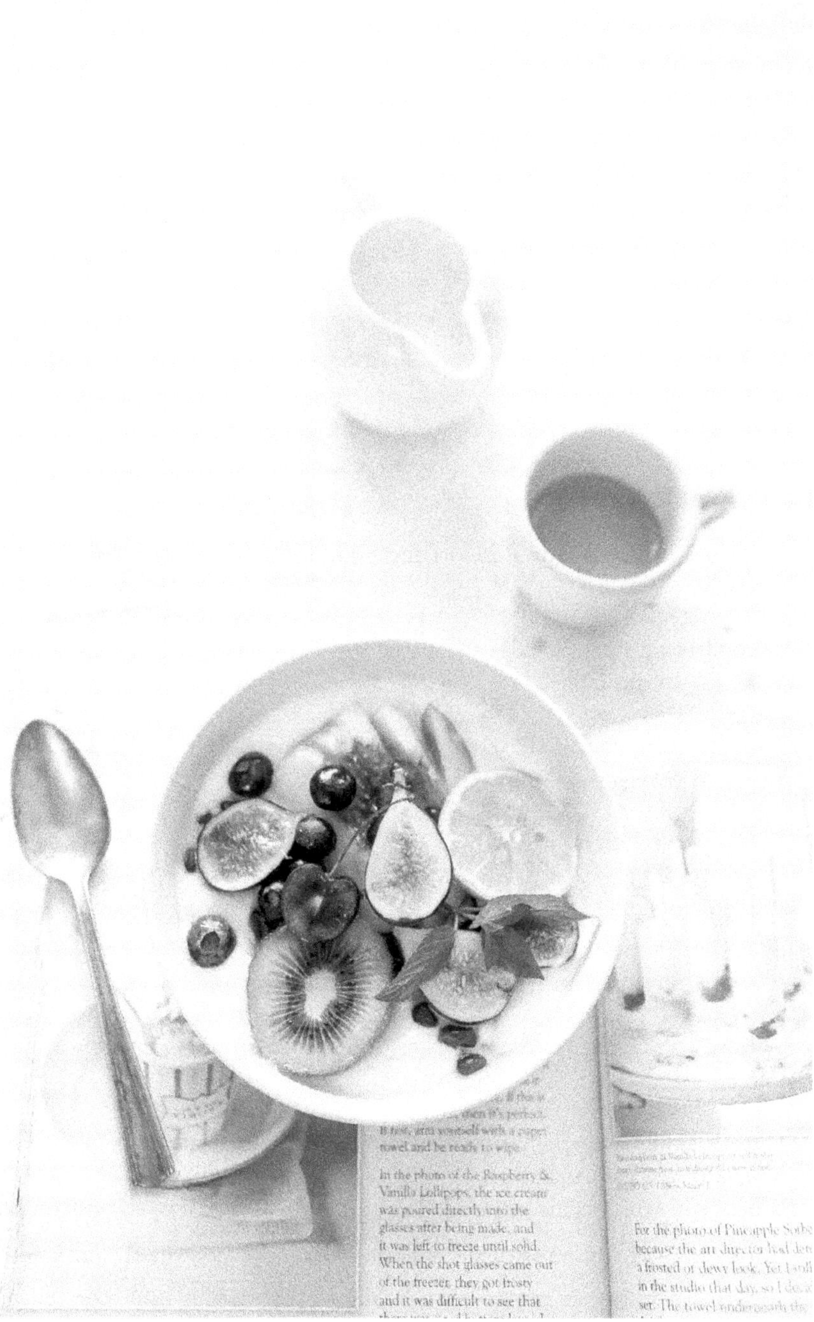
towel and be ready to wipe.
In the photo of the Raspberry &
Vanilla Lollipops, the ice cream
was poured directly into the
glasses after being made, and
it was left to freeze until solid.
When the shot glasses came out
of the freezer, they got frosty
and it was difficult to see that

Breakfasts

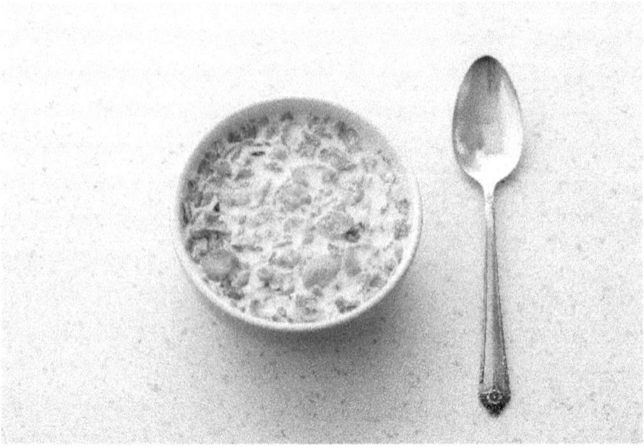

1 Vegetable Rice

Preparation time: 7 minutesCooking time: 15 minutes Servings: 4
Ingredients:

½ cup brown rice, rinsed1 cup water
½ teaspoon dried basil

1 small onion, chopped2 tablespoons raisins
5 ounces frozen peas, thawed

½ cup pecan halves, toasted

1 medium carrot, cut into matchsticks 4 green onions, cut into 1-inch pieces1 tablespoon olive oil
½ teaspoon salt or to taste

½ teaspoon crushed red chili flakes or to tasteGround pepper or to taste
Directions:

Place a small saucepan with water over medium heat. When it begins to boil, add rice and basil. Stir.
When it again begins to boil, lower the heat and cover with a lid.

Cook for 15 minutes until all the water is absorbed and rice is

cooked. Add more water if you think the rice is not cooked well. Meanwhile, place a skillet over medium high heat. Add carrots, raisins and onions and sauté until the vegetables are crisp as well astender.

Stir in the peas, salt, pepper and chili flakes.Add pecans and rice and stir.

Serve.

Nutrition: Calories 305, Fats 13 g, Carbohydrates 41 g, Proteins 8 g

2 Courgette Risotto

Preparation: 10 minutesCooking: 5 minutes Servings: 8
Ingredients:

2 tablespoons olive oil 4 cloves garlic, finely chopped

1.5 pounds Arborio rice6 tomatoes, chopped
2 teaspoons chopped rosemary

6 courgettes, finely diced

1 ¼ cups peas, fresh or frozen12 cups hot vegetable stock
1 cup chopped

Salt to taste

Freshly ground pepperDirections:
Place a large heavy bottomed pan over medium heat. Add oil. When

the oil is heated, add onion and sauté until translucent.Stir in the tomatoes and cook until soft.
Next stir in the rice and rosemary. Mix well.

Add half the stock and cook until dry. Stir frequently.Add remaining stock and cook for 3-4 minutes.

Add courgette and peas and cook until rice is tender. Add salt and pepper to taste.

Stir in the basil. Let it sit for 5 minutes.

Nutrition: Calories 406, Fats 5 g, Carbohydrates 82 g, Proteins 14 g

3 Country Breakfast Cereal

Preparation Time: 5 minutesCooking time: 40 minutes Servings: 6
Ingredients:

1 cup brown rice, uncooked

½ cup raisins, seedless1 tsp cinnamon, ground
¼ Tbsp peanut butter2 ¼ cups water Honey, to taste
Nuts, toastedDirections:
Combine rice, butter, raisins, and cinnamon in a saucepan. Add 2 ¼ cups water. Bring to boil.

Simmer covered for 40 minutes until rice is tender. Fluff with fork. Add honey and nuts to taste.
Nutrition: Calories 160 Carbohydrates 34 g Fats 1.5 g Protein 3 g

4 Root Vegetable Hash With Avocado Crème

Preparation time: 25 mCooking time: 10 m Ingredients:
1/2 c onion, diced1 T vegan butter
1 cloves garlic, minced

1 c sweet potatoes, diced1 c turnips, diced
1 c broccoli florets, diced2 vegan sausages, diced
1 c collard greens, chopped
1/2 tsp sea salt1 tsp cumin
1/2 tsp black pepper

1/4 – 1/2c vegetable stock 1/4 c fresh cilantro, chopped 1 medium avocado
1 T balsamic vinegar1/4 c cashews Directions:
Melt and hest the butter in a skillet. Add onion and garlic and sauté until they are translucent about 5 minutes.

Add sweet potatoes and turnips stir to match. Cook for 5-8 minutes.

Add the broccoli and vegetables. Continue cooking until it turns light green and start to soften for 5 to 8 minutes.

Add the roasted field, salt, pepper, cumin, coriander, and vinegar. Reduce the heat and get it cooked until the meat is hot and the flavors melt.

Mix the avocado, cashews, and vegetable broth in a blender until smooth.

Plate and serve with a spoonful of avocado cream on top. Garnish with more cilantro.

Nutrition: 19 g fat 30 g of carbohydrates 17 g protein 7 g sugar 691 mg sodium

5 Warm Maple and Cinnamon Quinoa

Preparation time: 5 minutesCooking time: 15 minutes Servings: 4
Ingredients

1 cup unsweetened nondairy milk1 cup water
1 cup quinoa, rinsed

1 teaspoon cinnamon

¼ Cup chopped pecans or other nuts or seeds, such as chia,sunflower seeds, or almonds

2 tablespoons pure maple syrup or agaveDirections:
In a medium saucepan over medium-high heat, bring the almond milk, water, and quinoa to a boil. Lower the heat to medium-low and cover. Simmer until the liquid is mostly absorbed and the quinoa softens, about 15 minutes.

Turn off the heat and allow to sit, covered, for 5 minutes. Stir in the cinnamon, pecans, and syrup. Serve hot.

6 Warm Quinoa Breakfast Bowl

Preparation time: 5 minutesCooking time: 0 minutes Servings: 4
Ingredients

3 cups freshly cooked quinoa

1 ⅓ cups unsweetened soy or almond milk2 bananas, sliced
1 cup raspberries

1 cup blueberries

½ Cup chopped raw walnuts

¼ Cup maple syrupDirections:
Divide the Ingredients among 4 bowls, starting with a base of ¾ cup

quinoa,⅓cupmilk,½banana,¼cupraspberries,¼ cup blueberries, and 2 tablespoons walnuts.

Drizzle 1 tablespoon of maple syrup over the top of each bowl.

7 Banana Bread Rice Pudding

Preparation time: 5 minutesCooking time: 50 minutes Servings: 4
Ingredients 1cup brown rice1½ cups water
1½ cups nondairy milk

3 tablespoons sugar (omit if using a sweetened nondairy milk)2 teaspoons pumpkin pie spice or ground cinnamon
2 bananas

3 tablespoons chopped walnuts or sunflower seeds (optional)Directions
In a medium pot, combine the rice, water, milk, sugar, and pumpkin

pie spice. Bring to a boil over high heat, turn the heat to low, and cover the pot. Simmer, stirring occasionally, until the rice is soft and the liquid is absorbed. White rice takes about 20 minutes; brown rice takes about 50 minutes.

Smash the bananas and stir them into the cooked rice. Serve toppedwith walnuts (if using). Leftovers will keep refrigerated in an airtight container for up to 5 days.

Nutrition: calories: 479; protein: 9g; total fat: 13g; saturated fat: 1g; carbohydrates: 86g; fiber: 7g

8 Breakfast Smoothie

Preparation: 10 minutesCooking: 0 minute Servings: 2
Ingredients:

½ cup strawberries ½ cup mango, sliced

½ banana, sliced ½ cup coconut milk

1 tablespoon cashew butter 1 tablespoon ground chia seeds Directions: ut all the ingredients in a blender.Pulse until smooth. Refrigerate overnight.

Nutrition: Calories: 299 Total fat: 14.5g Saturated fat: 4.2g Sodium: 64mg Potassium: 599mg Carbohydrates: 42.4g Fiber: 8.5g Sugar: 23g Protein: 5.3g

9 Yogurt with Beets & Raspberries

Preparation: 5 minutesCooking 0 minute Servings: 1
Ingredients:

1 cup soy yogurt

½ cup beets, cooked and sliced1 tablespoon raspberry jam
1 tablespoon almonds, sliveredDirections:
Mix all the ingredients in a glass jar with lid.Sprinkle the almonds on top. Refrigerate for up to 2 days.

Nutrition: Calories: 281 Total fat: 7.3g Saturated fat: 2.7g Cholesterol: 15mg Sodium: 237mg Potassium: 882mg Carbohydrates: 40.2g Fiber: 2.5g Sugar: 36g

10 Curry Oatmeal

Preparation Time: 10 minutesCooking Time: 0 minute Servings: 3
Ingredients:

1 tablespoon pure peanut butter

½ cup rolled oats

½ cup coconut milk

½ teaspoon curry powder1 teaspoon tamari
¼ cup cooked kale

1 tablespoon cilantro, chopped

2 tablespoons tomatoes, choppedDirections:
Mix all the ingredients except the kale, cilantro and tomatoes.Transfer to a glass jar with lid.
Refrigerate for up to 5 days.

Top with the remaining ingredients when ready to serve.

Nutrition: Calories: 307 Total fat: 13.8g Saturated fat: 4g Cholesterol:12mg Sodium: 467mg Potassium: 890mg Carbohydrates: 34.1g Fiber: 3g Sugar: 2g Protein: 10.1g

11 Peanut Butter Granola

Preparation time: 10 minutesCooking time: 47 minutes Servings: 04
Ingredients:

Nonstick spray4 cups oats
⅓ cup of cocoa powder

¾ cup peanut butter

⅓ cup maple syrup ⅓ cup avocado oil

1½ teaspoons vanilla extract

½ cup cocoa nibs

6 ounces dark chocolate, choppedDirections:
Preheat your oven to 300 degrees F. Spray a baking sheet with cooking spray.In a medium saucepan add oil, maple syrup, and peanut butter.

Cook for 2 minutes on medium heat, stirring. Add the oats and cocoa powder, mix well.
Spread the coated oats on the baking sheet.

Bake for 45 minutes, occasionally stirring.

Garnish with dark chocolate, cocoa nibs, and peanut butter.Serve.

Nutrition:Calories134TotalFat4.7gSaturatedFat0.6gCholesterol 124mg
Sodium 1 mg Total Carbs 54.1 g Fiber 7 g ugar
3.3 g Protein 6.2 g

Soups, Salads, and Sides

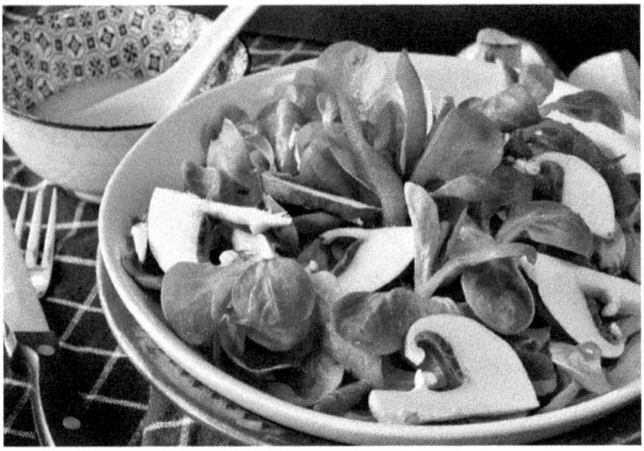

12 Rainbow Orzo Salad

Preparation time: 10 minutesCooking time: 20 minutes Servings: 1
Ingredients:

1 chopped onion

25g grated feta cheese2 sliced bell peppers

1 tablespoon olive oil6 sliced tomatoes

2 tablespoons chopped basil25g orzo pasta
Directions:

Preheat the oven at 350f temperature. Prepare a baking sheet and place the onion and bell peppers and drizzle half olive oil. Bake it for around 15 minutes. Add tomatoes on it and bake for an additional 5 minutes. Meanwhile, cook the orzo according to the given directions on the pack and cool it. Now toss it with the baked vegetables and top it with cheese, basil and remaining oil and serve it.

Nutrition: Carbohydrates 52g, protein 13g, fats 18g, calories 422, sugar 30g.

13 Broccoli Pasta Salad

Preparation time: 15 minutesChilling time: 30 minutes Servings: 12
Ingredients:

1-pound cooked pasta2 diced broccoli florets1 chopped onion
1 cup grated cheese

12 ounce cooked and finely chopped bacon

¾ teaspoon salt

¾ teaspoon ground black pepper1 cup mayonnaise
Directions:

Take a bowl and mix all the ingredients until all of them combined well. Cover it with the plastic wrap and place it in the refrigerator for at least 30 minutes and serve it. You can keep it in the refrigerator for3 days.

Nutrition: Carbohydrates 36g, protein 14g, fats 29g, calories 461.

14 Eggplant & Roasted Tomato Farro Salad

Preparation time: 1 hour Cooking time: 1 hour 30 minutes
Servings: 3

Ingredients:

4 small eggplants

1 ½ cups chopped cherry tomatoes

¾ cup uncooked faro1 tablespoon olive oil1 minced garlic clove
½ cup rinsed and drained chickpeas1 tablespoon basil
1 tablespoon arugula

½ teaspoon salt and ground black pepper1 tablespoon vinegar
½ cup toasted pine nuts

Directions:

Preheat the oven at 300f temperature and prepare a baking sheet. Place cherry tomatoes on the baking liner and drizzle olive oil, salt, and black pepper on it and bake it for 30 to 35 minutes. Cook thefaro in the salted water for 30 to 40 minutes. Slice the eggplant and salt it and leave it for 30 minutes. After that, rinse it with water and dry it kitchen towel. Now peeled and sliced the eggplants. Now place these slices on the baking liner and season it with salt, pepper and

olive oil. Bake it for 15 to 20 minutes in the preheated oven at the 450f temperature. Flip the sides of eggplant and bake it for anadditional 15 to 20 minutes. Bake the pine nuts for 5 minutes and sauté the garlic. Now mix all the ingredients in a bowl and serve it.

Nutrition: Carbohydrates 37g, protein 9g, fats 25g, calories 399.

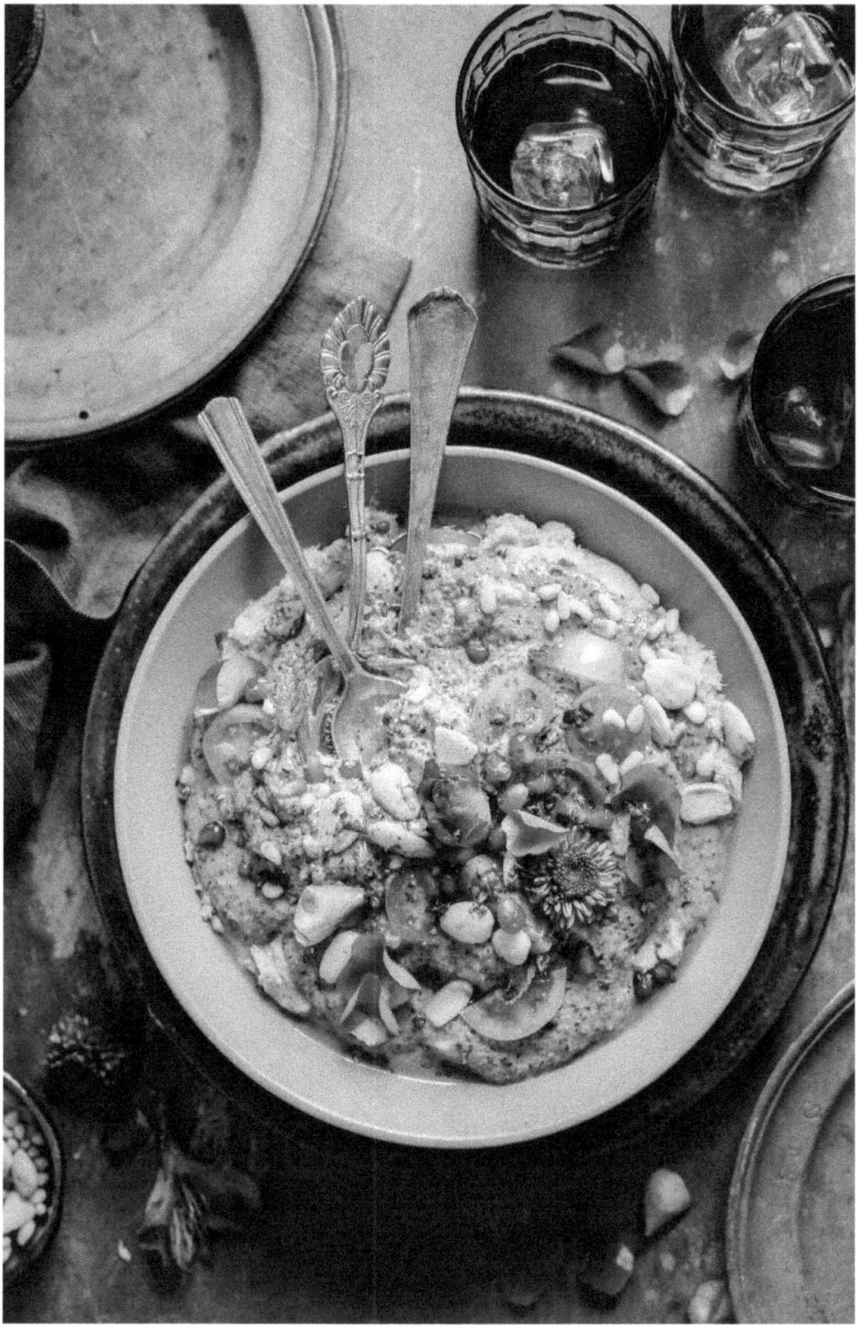

Entrées

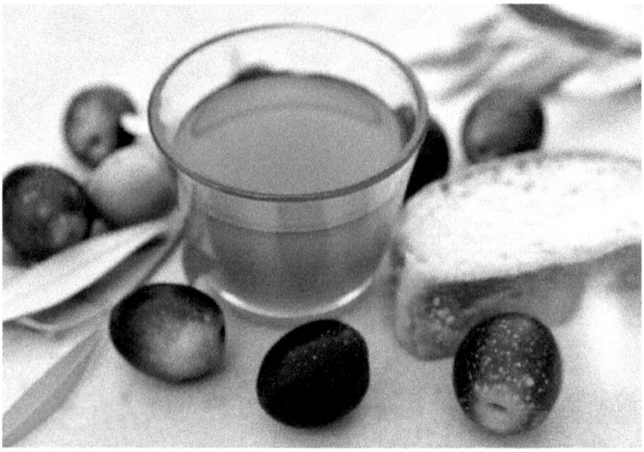

15 Garlicky Kale Chips

Preparation time: 1 hour and 30 minCooking time: 1 hour
Servings: 2

Ingredients:

4 cloves garlic1 cup olive oil
8 to 10 cups fresh kale, chopped

1 tablespoon of garlic-flavored olive oil

½ teaspoon garlic salt

½ teaspoon pepper

1 pinch red pepper flakes (optional)Directions:
Peel and crush the garlic clove and place it in a small jar with a lid.

Pour the olive oil over the top, cover tightly and shake. This will keep in the refrigerator for several days. When you're ready to use it, strain out the garlic and retain the oil.

Preheat the oven to 175 degrees, Fahrenheit.

Spread out the kale on a baking sheet and drizzle with the olive oil. Sprinkle with garlic salt, pepper and red pepper flakes.

Bake for an hour, remove from the oven and let the chips cool. Store in an airtight container if you don't plan to eat them right away.

16 Hummus-stuffed Baby Potatoes

Preparation time: 30 minutesCooking time: 30 minutes Servings: 2
Ingredients:

12 small red potatoes, walnut-sized or slightly largerHummus
2 green onions, thinly sliced

¼ teaspoon paprika, for garnishDirections:
Place two to three inches of water in a saucepan, set a steamer inside and bring the water to a boil.

Place the whole potatoes in the steamer basket and steam for about 20 minutes or until soft. Keep the pan from boiling dry by adding additional hot water as needed.

Dump the potatoes into a colander and run cold water over them until they can be handled.

Cut each potato open and scoop out most of the pulp, leaving the skin and a thin layer of potato intact.

Mix the hummus with most of the green onions (keep enough for garnish) and spoon a little into the area where the potato has been scooped out.

Sprinkle each filled potato half with paprika and serve.

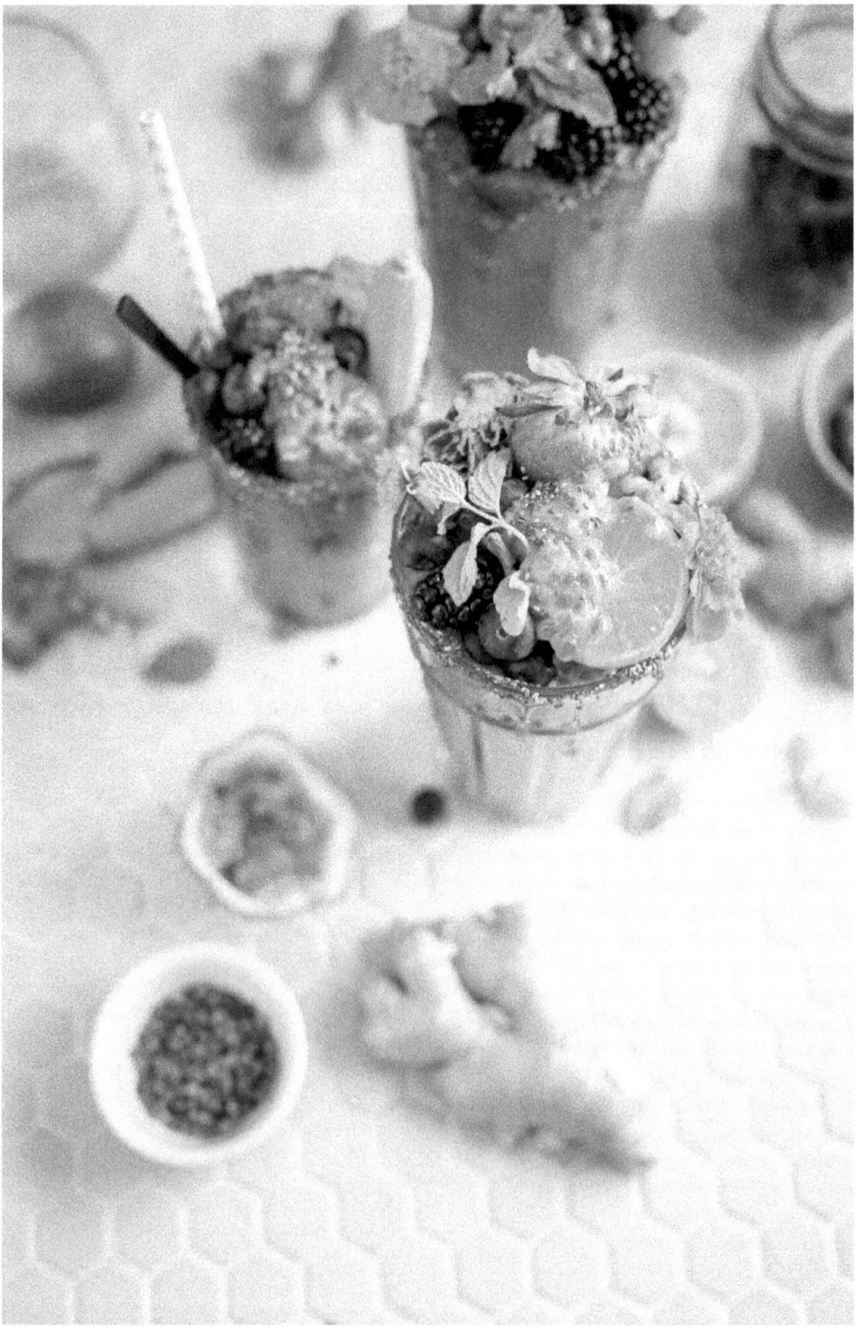

Smoothies and Beverages

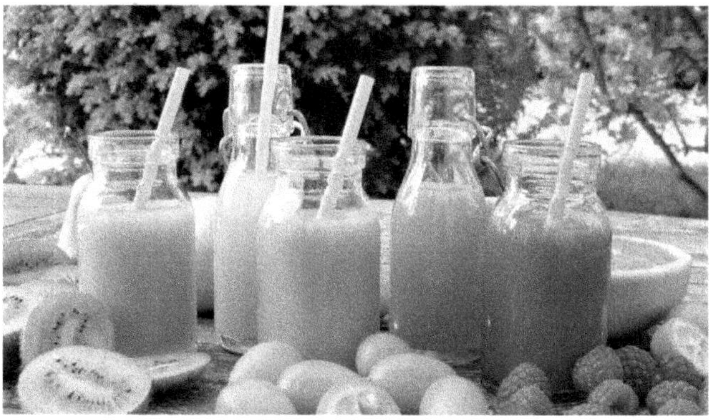

17 Ultimate Mulled Wine

Preparation: 35 minutesCooking: 30 minutes Servings: 6
Ingredients:

1 cup of cranberries, fresh2 oranges, juiced
1 tablespoon of whole cloves

2 cinnamon sticks, each about 3 inches long1 tablespoon of star anise
1/3 cup of honey 8 fluid ounce of apple cider

8 fluid ounce of cranberry juice24 fluid ounce of red wine Directions:
Using a 4 quarts slow cooker, add all the ingredients and stirproperly.

Cover it with the lid, then plug in the slow cooker and cook it for 30 minutes on thee high heat setting or until it gets warm thoroughly.

When done, strain the wine and serve right away.

Nutrition: Calories:202 Cal, Carbohydrates:25g, Protein:0g, Fats:0g, Fiber:0g.

18 Pleasant Lemonade

Preparation time: 3 hours and 15 minutesCooking time: 3 hours
Servings: 10 servings

Ingredients:

Cinnamon sticks for serving2 cups of coconut sugar 1/4 cup of honey
3 cups of lemon juice. fresh32 fluid ounce of water Directions:
Using a 4-quarts slow cooker, place all the ingredients except for the cinnamon sticks and stir properly.

Cover it with the lid, then plug in the slow cooker and cook it for 3 hours on the low heat setting or until it is heated thoroughly.

When done, stir properly and serve with the cinnamon sticks.

Nutrition: Calories:146 Cal, Carbohydrates:34g, Protein:0g, Fats:0g, Fiber:0g.

19 Pineapple, Banana & Spinach Smoothie

Preparation: 10 MinutesCooking: 0 minute Servings: 1
Ingredients:

½ cup almond milk ¼ cup soy yogurt1 cup spinach
1 cup banana

1 cup pineapple chunks1 tbsp. chia seeds Direction:
Add all the ingredients in a blender.Blend until smooth.
Chill in the refrigerator before serving.

Nutrition: Calories 297, Total Fat 6 g, Saturated Fat 1 g, Cholesterol4 mg Sodium 145 mg, Total Carbohydrate 54 g, Dietary Fiber 10 g Protein 13g, Total Sugars 29g, Potassium 1038 mg

20 White Chocolate Pudding

Preparation Time: 4 hours 20 minutes

Servings: 4Ingredients
3 tbsp flax seed + 9 tbsp water 3 tbsp cornstarch ¼ tbsp salt 1 cup cashew cream 2 ½ cups almond milk
½ pure date sugar 1 tbsp vanilla caviar
6 oz unsweetened white chocolate chips Whipped coconut cream for topping
Sliced bananas and raspberries for topping

Directions

In a small bowl, mix the flax seed powder with water and allow thickening for 5 minutes to make the flax egg.

In a large bowl, whisk the cornstarch and salt, and then slowly mix in the in the cashew cream until smooth. Whisk in the flax egg until well combined.

Pour the almond milk into a pot and whisk in the date sugar. Cook over medium heat while frequently stirring until the sugar dissolves. Reduce the heat to low and simmer until steamy and bubbly around the edges.

Pour half of the almond milk mixture into the flax egg mix, whisk well and pour this mixture into the remaining milk content in the pot. Whisk continuously until well combined.

Bring the new mixture to a boil over medium heat while still frequently stirring and scraping all the corners of the pot, 2 minutes.

Turn the heat off, stir in the vanilla caviar, then the white chocolate chips until melted. Spoon the mixture into a bowl, allow cooling for 2 minutes, cover with plastic wraps making sure to press the plastic onto the surface of the pudding, and refrigerate for 4 hours.

Remove the pudding from the fridge, take off the plastic wrap and whip for about a minute.

Spoon the dessert into serving cups, swirl some coconut whipping cream on top, and top with the bananas and raspberries. Enjoy immediately.

Nutritional info per serving

Calories 654 | Fats 47.9g| Carbs 52.1g | Protein 7.3g

21 Ambrosia Salad With Pecans

Preparation Time: 15 minutes + 1 hour chillingServings: 4
These are the ingredients that inflict anguish if skipped at the celebration plate.

Ingredients

1 cup pure coconut cream

½ tsp vanilla extract

2 medium bananas, peeled and cut into chunks 1 ½ cups unsweetened coconut flakes
4 tbsp toasted pecans, chopped

1 cup pineapple tidbits, drained

1 (11 oz) can mandarin oranges, drained

¾ cup maraschino cherries, stems removedDirections
In medium bowl, mix the coconut cream and vanilla extract until well combined.

In a larger bowl, combine the bananas, coconut flakes, pecans,pineapple, oranges, and cherries until evenly distributed.

Pour on the coconut cream mixture and fold well into the salad. Chill in the refrigerator for 1 hour and serve afterwards.
Nutritional info per serving

Calories 648 | Fats 36g| Carbs 85.7g | Protein 6.6g

22 Peanut Butter Blossom Biscuits

Preparation: 15 minutes + 1 hour chillingServings: 4
Ingredients

1 tbsp flax seed powder + 3 tbsp water

1 cup pure date sugar + more for dusting

½ cup creamy peanut butter1 tsp vanilla extract

1 ¾ cup whole-wheat flour1 tsp baking soda
¼ tsp salt ¼ cup unsweetened chocolate chipsDirections
In a small bowl, mix the flax seed powder with water and allow thickening for 5 minutes to make the flax egg.

In a medium bowl using an electric mixer, whisk the date sugar, plant butter, and peanut butter until light and fluffy.

Mix in the flax egg and vanilla until well combined. Add the flour, baking soda, salt, and whisk well again.

Fold in the chocolate chips, cover the bowl with a plastic wrap, and refrigerate for 1 hour. After, preheat the oven to 375 F and line a baking sheet with parchment paper.

Use a cookie sheet to scoop mounds of the batter onto the sheet with 1-inch intervals. Bake in the oven for 9 to 10 minutes or until golden brown and slightly cracked on top. Remove the cookies from the oven, cool for 3 minutes, roll in some date sugar, and serve. Nutritional info per serving Calories 839 | Fats 52.5g| Carbs 77.9g | Protein 21.1g

23 Chocolate & Almond Butter Barks

Preparation Time: 35 minutesServings: 4
Chewy fluffy almonds is equal to delicious almond bark, handmade dairy-free chocolate bars!Ingredients
1/3 cup coconut oil, melted

¼ cup almond butter, melted

2 tbsp unsweetened coconut flakes.1 tsp pure maple syrup
A pinch ground rock salt

¼ cup unsweetened cocoa nibsDirections
Line a baking tray with baking paper and set aside.

In a medium bowl, mix the coconut oil, almond butter, coconut flakes, maple syrup, and then fold in the rock salt and cocoa nibs.

Pour and spread the mixture on the baking sheet, chill in therefrigerator for 20 minutes or until firm.

Remove the dessert, break into shards and enjoy immediately. Preserve extras in the refrigerator.
Nutritional info per serving

Calories 279 | Fats 28.1g| Carbs 8.6g | Protein 4.4g

Snacks and Desserts

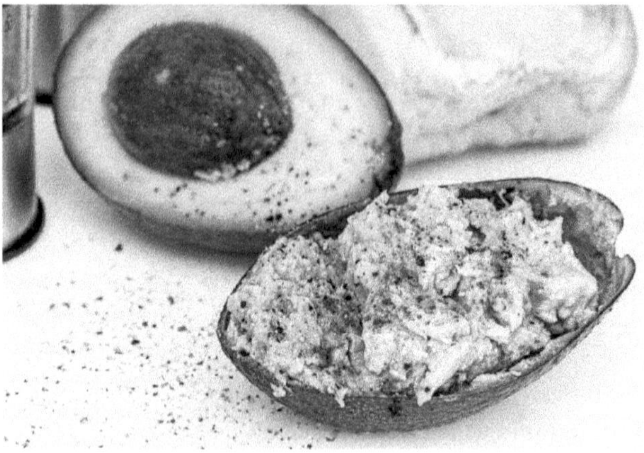

24 Raspberries & Cream Ice Cream

Preparation time: 5 minsCooking time: 0 mins Servings: 4
Ingredients

2 Cups Raspberries 8 Oz. Coconut Cream
2 Tbsps. Coconut Flour

1 Tsp Maple Syrup

4-8 Raspberries For FillingDirections
Mix all ingredients in food processor and blend until well combined.

Spoon mixture into silicone mold and with raspberries and freeze for about 4 hours.

Remove balls from freezer and pop them out of the molds. Serve immediately and enjoy!
Nutrition: Protein: 5% 12 kcal Fat: 69% 170 kcal Carbohydrates: 26% 63 kcal

25 Healthy Chocolate Mousse

Preparation time: 5 minsCooking time: 0 mins Servings: 2
Ingredients

1/2 Cup Coconut Milk1 Tsp. Maple Syrup
1-3 Tbsps. Cocoa Powder

Pinch Instant Coffee

2 Tbsps. Coconut CreamBlackberries For ToppingDirections
Heat up coconut milk and maple syrup until it just begins to simmer.Add cocoa and coffee in milk mixture.
Add cream to same mixture and whip until relatively stiff peaks form. Transfer to a serving glass.
Chill the mousse in freezer for 2-3 hours.

Top with some berries and spoon of coconut cream.Enjoy!
Nutrition: Protein: 3% 7 kcal Fat: 83% 163 kcal Carbohydrates: 13%

26 kcal

26 Coconut Rice With Mangos

Preparation time: 15 minsCooking time: 40 mins Servings: 6
Ingredients

2 Cups Coconut Milk

1-1/2 Cups Coconut Flakes1/4 Cup Maple Syrup
1 Mango SlicedDirections
Heat saucepan over high heat.

Add coconut milk and bring it to boil. Stir in coconut flakes and maple syrup.
Cover and cook on low heat for about 15 minutes or until liquid is completely dried.

Pour coconut rice in plate.

Serve with mango slice and enjoy.

Nutrition: Protein: 3% 8 kcal Fat: 69% 185 kcal Carbohydrates: 28% 75 kcal

27 Honey Peanut Butter

Preparation time: 10 minutesCooking time: 0 minutes Servings: 6
Ingredients

1 cup peanut butter

3/4 cup honey extracted1/2 cup ground peanuts1 tsp ground cinnamon
Directions:
Add all ingredients into your fast-speed blender, and blend untilsmooth.

Keep refrigerated.

28 Mediterranean Marinated Olives

Preparation time: 10 minutesCooking time: 0 minutes Servings: 2
Ingredients

24 large olives, black, green, Kalamata1/2 cup extra-virgin olive oil
4 cloves garlic, thinly sliced 2 Tbsp fresh lemon juice

2 tsp coriander seeds, crushed1/2 tsp crushed red pepper
1 tsp dried thyme1 tsp dried rosemary, crushed Salt and ground pepper to taste

Directions:
Place olives and all remaining ingredients in a large container or bag, and shake to combine well.

Cover and refrigerate to marinate overnight.Serve.
Keep refrigerated.

29 Nut Butter & Dates Granola

Preparation: 1 hour Cooking: 55 minutesServings: 8
Ingredients

3 cups rolled oats

2 cups dates, pitted and chopped1 cup flaked or shredded coconut1/2 cup wheat germ
1/4 cup soy milk powder 1/2 cup almonds chopped 3/4 cup honey strained
1/2 cup almond butter (plain, unsalted) softened 1/4 cup peanut butter softened
Directions:

Preheat oven to 300F.

Add all ingredients into a food processor and pulse until roughly combined.

Spread mixture evenly into greased 10 x 15-inch baking pan.Bake for 45 to 55 minutes.
Stir mixture several times during baking.

Remove from the oven and cool completely.Store in a covered glass jar.

30 Hazelnut & Maple Chia Crunch

Preparation Time: 30 MinutesCooking Time: 5 Minutes Servings: 2
Ingredients:

Chia Seeds (.25 C.)

Olive Oil (1 t.)

Maple Syrup (.50 C.)Hazelnuts (1.25 C.) Salt (to Taste) Directions:
To begin this recipe, start by heating a pan over medium heat. Once warm, place the olive oil and maple in and bring to a boil.

Once boiling, stir in your hazelnuts and cook on high for a minute or two. After this time passes, add in the chia seeds and salt and cook for another three minutes.

Now, turn the heat down to low and begin crushing the hazelnuts in the pan before pouring onto a lined cookie sheet. At this point, try to spread the mixture evenly across the pan and then place it in the freezer for 15 minutes.

Once the mixture has completely cooled, chop the ingredients into clusters and enjoy.

Nutrition: Calories: 330 Proteins: 3g Carbs: 60g Fats: 11g

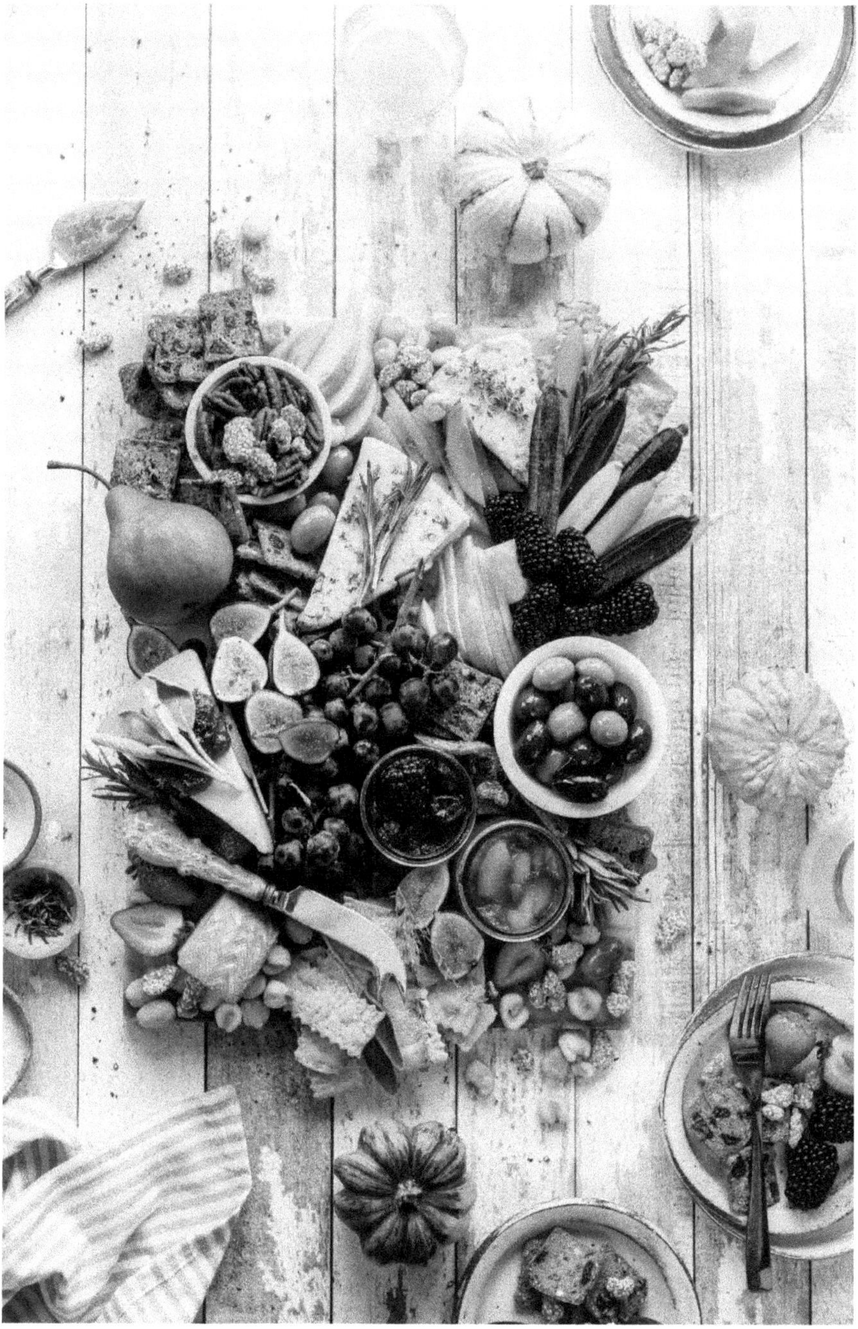

Dinner Recipes

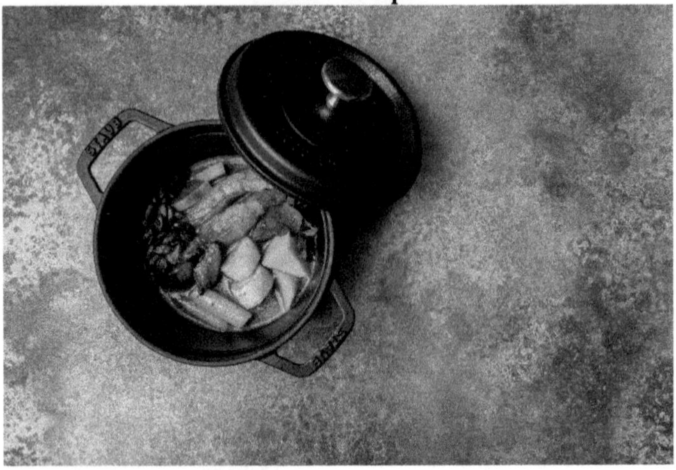

31 Butternut Squash Steak

Preparation Time: 30 min.Cooking Time: 50 min.
Servings: 4

Ingredients:

2 tbsp. coconut yogurt

½ t. sweet paprika

1 ¼ c. low-sodium vegetable broth

1 sprig thyme

1 finely chopped garlic clove1 big thinly sliced shallot

1 tbsp. margarine

2 tbsp. olive oil, extra virginSalt and pepper to liking Directions:
Bring the oven to 375 heat setting.

Cut the squash, lengthwise, into 4 steaks.

Carefully core one side of each squash with a paring knife in a crosshatch pattern.

Using a brush, coat with olive oil each side of the steak then season generously with salt and pepper.

In an oven-safe, non-stick skillet, bring 2 tablespoons of olive oil to a warm temperature.

Place the steaks on the skillet with the cored side down and cook at medium temperature until browned, approximately 5 minutes.

Flip and repeat on the other side for about 3 minutes.

Place the skillet into the oven to roast the squash for 7 minutes.

Take out from the oven, placing on a plate and covering withaluminum foil to keep warm.

Using the previously used skillet, add thyme, garlic, and shallot, cooking at medium heat. Stir frequently for about 2 minutes.

Add brandy and cook for an additional minute.

Next, add paprika and whisk the mixture together for 3 minutes. Add in the yogurt seasoning with salt and pepper.
Plate the steaks and spoon the sauce over the top.

Garnish with parsley and enjoy!

Nutrition: Calories: 300 | Carbohydrates: 46 g | Proteins: 5.3 g | Fats: 10.6g

32 Eggplant & mushrooms in peanut sauce

Preparation time 32 minutesCooking time: 10 minutes Servings: 6
Ingredients:

4 Japanese eggplants cut into 1-inch thick round slices

3/4 pounds of shiitake mu shrooms, stems discarded, halved3 tablespoons smooth peanut butter
2 1/2 tablespoons rice vinegar1 1/2 tablespoons soy sauce
1 1/2 tablespoons, peeled, fresh ginger, finely grated1 1/2 tablespoons light brown sugar
Coarse salt to taste

3 scallions, cut into 2-inch lengths, thinly sliced lengthwiseDirection:
Placetheeggplantsandmushroominasteamer.Steamthe eggplant and mushrooms until tender. Transfer to a bowl.

To a small bowl, add peanut butter and vinegar and whisk.

Add rest of the ingredients and whisk well. Add this to the bowl of eggplant slices. Add scallions and mix well.

Serve hot.

33 Cassoulet

Preparation time: 35 minutes Cooking time: 1 hr and 30 minutesServings: 4

Protein content per serving: 22 gIngredients

¼ cup (60 ml) olive oil, divided

4 ounces (113 g) quit-the-cluck seitan, chopped1/3 of a smoky sausage, chopped

1½ cups (240 g) chopped onion

2 ounces (57 g) minced shiitake mushrooms

2 large carrots, peeled, sliced into ¼-inch (6 mm) rounds2 stalks celery, chopped

1½ cups (355 ml) vegetable broth, divided

1 teaspoon liquid smoke

3 cans (each 15 ounces, or 425 g) white beans of choice, drainedand rinsed

1 can (14.5 ounces, or 410 g) diced tomatoes, undrained

2 tablespoons (32 g) tomato paste 1 tablespoon (15 ml) tamari

1 tablespoon (18 g) no chicken bouillon paste, or 2 bouillon cubes, crumbled

2 tablespoons (8 g) minced fresh parsley2 teaspoons dried thyme

½ teaspoon dried rosemary salt and pepper2 cups (200 g) fresh bread crumbs

½ cup (40 g) panko crumbsDirection

Preheat the oven to 375°f (190°c, or gas mark 5).

Heat 1 tablespoon (15 ml) of olive oil in a large skillet over medium heat.

Add the seitan and sausage. Cook for 4 to 6 minutes, occasionally stirring, until browned. Transfer to a plate and set aside.

Add the onion and a pinch of salt to the same skillet. Cook for 5 to 7 minutes until translucent. Transfer to the same plate. Add the shiitakes, carrots, and celery to the skillet and cook for 2 minutes. Add 1 tablespoon (15 ml) vegetable broth and the liquid smoke.Cook for 2 to 3 minutes, stirring until the liquid is absorbed or evaporated.

Return the seitan and onions to the skillet and add the beans, tomatoes, tomato paste, tamari, bouillon, parsley, thyme, rosemary, and remaining broth. Cook for 3 to 4 minutes, stirring to combine.

Season with salt and pepper to taste and transfer to a large casserole pan.

Toss together the fresh bread crumbs, panko crumbs, and the remaining 3 tablespoons (45 ml) olive oil in a small bowl. Spread evenly over the bean mixture. Bake for 30 to 35 minutes until the crumbs are browned.

34 Double-garlic bean and vegetable soup

Preparation time: 25 minutesCooking time: 10 minutes Servings: 4
Protein content per serving: 21 gIngredients
1 tablespoon (15 ml) olive oil

1 teaspoon fine sea salt

1 (240 g) minced onion 5 cloves garlic, minced2 cups (220 g) chopped red potatoes
⅔ cup (96 g) sliced carrots

Protein content per serving cup (60 g) chopped celery 1 teaspoon italian seasoning blend
Protein content per serving teaspoon red pepper flakes, or to taste

Protein content per serving teaspoon celery seed 4 cups water (940 ml), divided
1 can (14.5 ounces, or 410 g) crushed tomatoes or tomato puree

1 head roasted garlic

2 tablespoons (30 g) prepared vegan pesto, plus more for garnish

2 cans (each 15 ounces, or 425 g) different kinds of white beans, drained and rinsed

Protein content per serving cup (50 g) 1-inch (2.5 cm) pieces green beans
Salt and pepper
Directions:

Heat the oil and salt in a large soup pot over medium heat. Add the onion, garlic, potatoes, carrots, and celery. Cook for 4 to 6 minutes, occasionally stirring, until the onions are translucent. Add the seasoning blend, red pepper flakes, and celery seed and stir for 2 minutes. Add 3 cups (705 ml) of the water and the crushed tomatoes.

Combine the remaining 1 cup (235 ml) water and the roasted garlicin a blender. Process until smooth. Add to the soup mixture andbring to a boil. Reduce the heat to simmer and cook for 30 minutes.

Stir in the pesto, beans, and green beans. Simmer for 15 minutes. Taste and adjust the seasonings. Serve each bowl with a dollop of pesto, if desired.

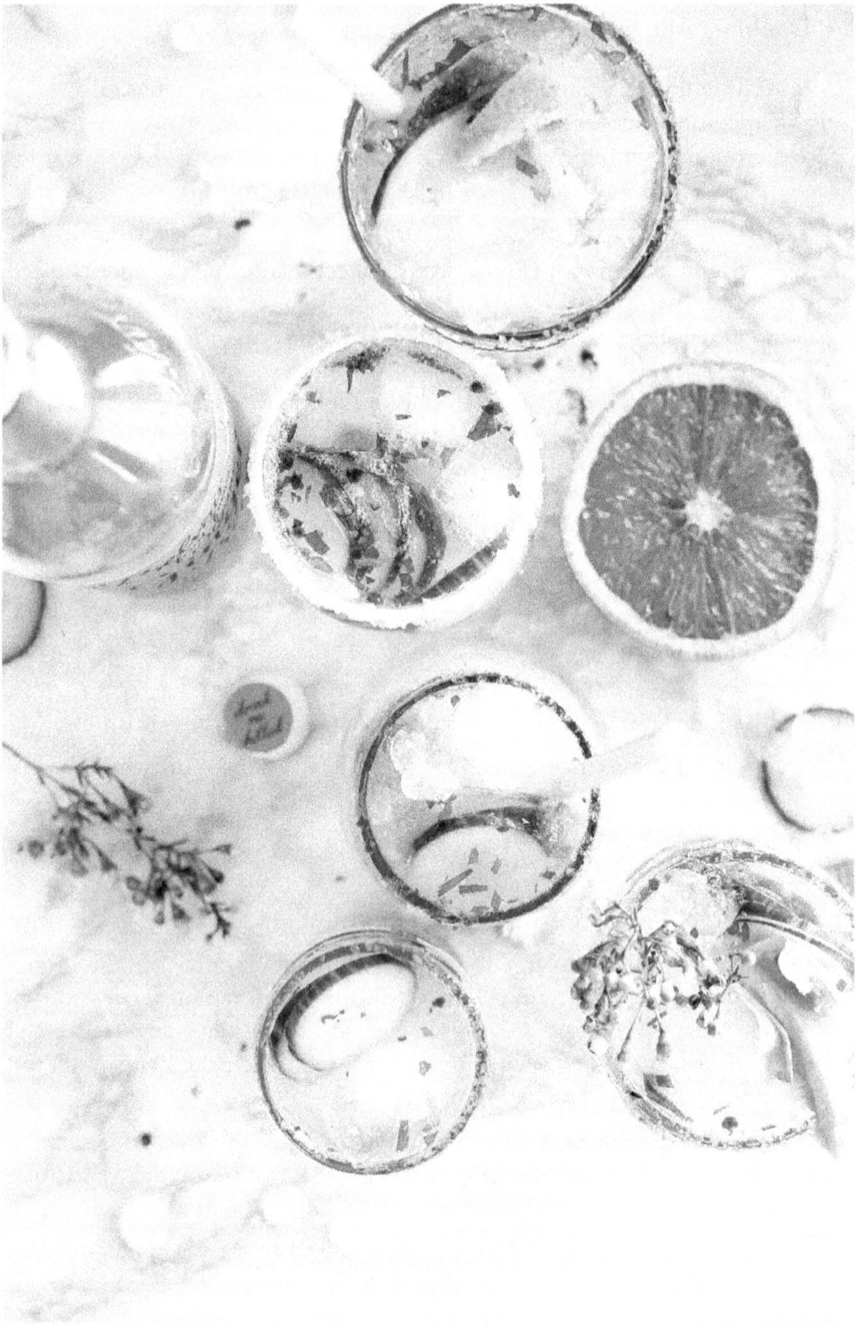

Lunch Recipes

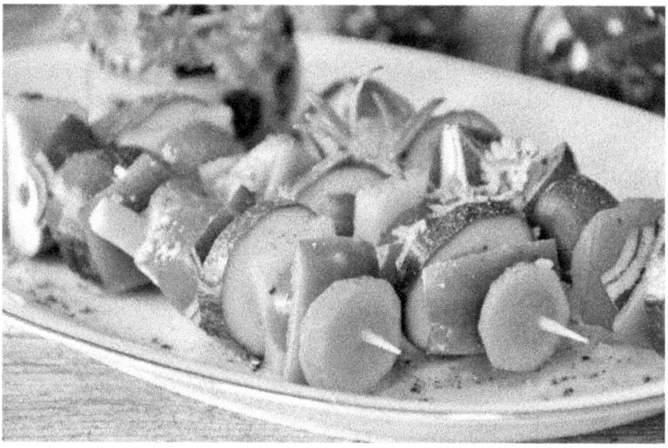

35 Breaded Tofu Steaks

Preparation Time: 10 minutesCooking Time: 12 minutes Serving: 4 Ingredients:

3 cups (750 grams) tofu, extra-firm, pressed4 tablespoons tomato paste

2 ½ tablespoons minced garlic

1 cup (236 grams) panko breadcrumbs and more as needed

½ teaspoon ground black pepper2 tablespoon maple syrup

2 tablespoon Dijon mustard

2 tablespoon soy sauce4 tablespoons olive oil 2 tablespoon water BBQ sauce for serving Directions:

Prepare the tofu steaks: pat dry tofu and then cut them into four slices.

Prepare the sauce: take a medium bowl, add garlic, black pepper, maple syrup, mustard, tomato paste, soy sauce, and water; stir until combined.

Take a shallow dish and place bread crumbs on it.

Working on one tofu steak at a time, first coat it with prepared sauce,then dredge it with bread crumbs until evenly coated and place it ona plate.

Repeat with the remaining tofu slices.

Take a frying pan, place it over medium heat, pour oil in it and when hot, place a tofu steak inside and cook for 4 to 6 minutes per side until golden brown and cooked.

Transfer tofu steak to a plate and repeat with the remaining tofu steaks.

Serve tofu steaks with the BBQ sauce.

Nutrition: 419.4 Cal; 23.9 g Fat; 3.9 g Saturated Fat; 33.3 g Carbs; 4.3 g Fiber; 22.8 g Protein; 3 g Sugar;

36 Quinoa Avocado Salad

Preparation Time: 15 minutesCooking Time: 4 minutes Servings: 4
Ingredients:

2 tablespoons balsamic vinegar

¼ cup cream

¼ cup buttermilk

5 tablespoons freshly squeezed lemon juice, divided1 clove garlic, grated
2 tablespoons shallot, mincedSalt and pepper to taste
2 tablespoons avocado oil, divided1 ¼ cups quinoa, cooked
2 heads endive, sliced

2 firm pears, sliced thinly2 avocados, sliced
¼ cup fresh dill, chopped

Direction

Combine the vinegar, cream, milk, 1 tablespoon lemon juice, garlic, shallot, salt and pepper in a bowl.

Pour 1 tablespoon oil into a pan over medium heat.Heat the quinoa for 4 minutes.

Transfer quinoa to a plate.

Toss the endive and pears in a mixture of remaining oil, remaining lemon juice, salt and pepper.

Transfer to a plate.

Toss the avocado in the reserved dressing.Add to the plate.
Top with the dill and quinoa.

Nutrition: Calories: 431 Total fat: 28.5g Saturated fat: 8g Cholesterol:13mg Sodium: 345mg Potassium: 779mg Carbohydrates: 42.7gFiber: 6g Sugar: 3g Protein: 6.6g

37 Roasted Sweet Potatoes

Preparation Time: 20 minutesCooking Time: 20 minutes Servings: 4
Ingredients:

2 potatoes, sliced into wedges 2 tablespoons olive oil, divided Salt and pepper to taste

1 red bell pepper, chopped

¼ cup fresh cilantro, chopped1 garlic, minced

2 tablespoons almonds, toasted and sliced

1 tablespoon lime juiceDirection

Preheat your oven to 425 degrees F. Toss the sweet potatoes in oil and salt.Transfer to a baking pan.

Roast for 20 minutes.

In a bowl, combine the red bell pepper, cilantro, garlic and almonds. In another bowl, mix the lime juice, remaining oil, salt and pepper.

Drizzle this mixture over the red bell pepper mixture. Serve sweet potatoes with the red bell pepper mixture.

Nutrition: Calories: 146 Total fat: 8.6g Saturated fat: 1.1g Sodium: 317mg Potassium: 380mg Carbohydrates: 16g Fiber: 2.9g Sugar: 5g Protein: 2.3g

38 Roasted Tomato Sandwich

This sandwich is full of fresh ingredients, many of which cannot be prepared ahead. But, when you simply have to prepare some lettuce, an avocado, or tomato, this is not a problem. You can still have an easy and quick meal. But, that doesn't mean you can't prepare any aspects of this sandwich ahead of time. If using homemade bread, you can prepare it at the beginning of the week and store it in the cold-storage box or icebox. You can also prepare the garlic aioli ahead of time and store it in a Mason jar in the fridge.

Preparation time: 30 minutesCooking Time: 25 minutes Servings: 2
Ingredients:

Sourdough bread – 4 slices

Tomatoes, large, cut into eight rounds – 2Avocado – 1
Sea salt – .25 teaspoon

Vegan mayonnaise – .25 cupGarlic, minced – 2 cloves
Juice of lemon fruit – 1 tablespoon Oregano, dried – .25 teaspoon Black ground pepper – .25 teaspoonOlive oil – 2 tablespoons
Fresh basil – .25 cup

Arugula – .25 cupDirections:
Begin by setting your electric cooker to Fahrenheit 350 degrees and

lining an aluminum sheet pan with kitchen parchment. Layout the sliced tomatoes on the sheet, and sprinkle them with part of the salt, oregano, and pepper, and allow them to roast until tender, about fifteen minutes.

Meanwhile, prepare the garlic aioli. Whisk together the mayonnaise, garlic, juice of lemon fruit, and some sea salt and pepper. Chill in the fridge until use.

Use a pastry brush and coat one side of each slice of bread with the olive oil. While doing this preheat a skillet over midway warmth. Once hot, toast the bread oil-side down until browned and thenremove them from the heat.

To prepare the sandwiches, lay out the bread, oil side down. On each slice spread the garlic aioli. On half of the slices cover with the roasted tomatoes, sliced avocado, basil, and arugula. Top these slices with their matched slice without toppings. Slice the sandwiches in half before serving.

Nutrition: Calories 525

39 Arugula and Artichokes Bowls

Preparation time: 5 minutesCooking time: 0 minutes Servings: 4
Ingredients:

1 cups baby arugula

¼ cup walnuts, chopped

1 cup canned artichoke hearts, drained and quartered 1 tablespoon balsamic vinegar

2 tablespoons cilantro, chopped

2 tablespoons olive oil

Salt and black pepper to the taste1 tablespoon lemon juice Directions:
In a bowl, combine the artichokes with the arugula, walnuts and the other ingredients, toss, divide into smaller bowls and serve for lunch.

Nutrition: calories 200, fat 2, fiber 1, carbs 5, protein 7

40 Minty arugula soup

Preparation time: 5 minutesCooking time: 10 minutes Servings: 4
Ingredients:

3 scallions, chopped 1 tablespoon olive oil
½ Cup coconut milk

2 cups baby arugula

2 tablespoons mint, chopped6 cups vegetable stock

2 tablespoons chives, chopped Salt and black pepper to the taste
Directions:

Heat up a pot with the oil over medium high heat, add the scallionsand sauté for 2 minutes.

Add the rest of the ingredients, toss, bring to a simmer and cook over medium heat for 8 minutes more.

Divide the soup into bowls and serve.

Nutrition: calories 200, fat 4, fiber 2, carbs 6, protein 10

41 Spinach and Broccoli Soup

Preparation time: 10 minutesCooking time: 20 minutes Servings: 4
Ingredients:

3 shallots, chopped 1 tablespoon olive oil
2 garlic cloves, minced

½ pound broccoli florets

½ pound baby spinach

Salt and black pepper to the taste4 cups veggie stock
1 teaspoon turmeric powder1 tablespoon lime juice Directions:
Heat up a pot with the oil over medium high heat, add the shallots and the garlic and sauté for 5 minutes.

Add the broccoli, spinach and the other ingredients, toss, bring to a simmer and cook over medium heat for 15 minutes.

Ladle into soup bowls and serve.

Nutrition: calories 150, fat 3, fiber 1, carbs 3, protein 7

42 Eggplant and Peppers Soup

Preparation time: 10 minutesCooking time: 40 minutes Servings: 4

Ingredients:

2 red bell peppers, chopped3 scallions, chopped

3 garlic cloves, minced2 tablespoon olive oil

Salt and black pepper to the taste

5 cups vegetable stock1 bay leaf

½ cup coconut cream

1 pound eggplants, roughly cubed 2 tablespoons basil, chopped

Directions:

Heat up a pot with the oil over medium heat, add the scallions andthe garlic and sauté for 5 minutes.

Add the peppers and the eggplants and sauté for 5 minutes more.

Add the remaining ingredients, toss, bring to a simmer, cook for 30 minutes, ladle into bowls and serve for lunch.

Nutrition: calories 180, fat 2, fiber 3, carbs 5, protein 10

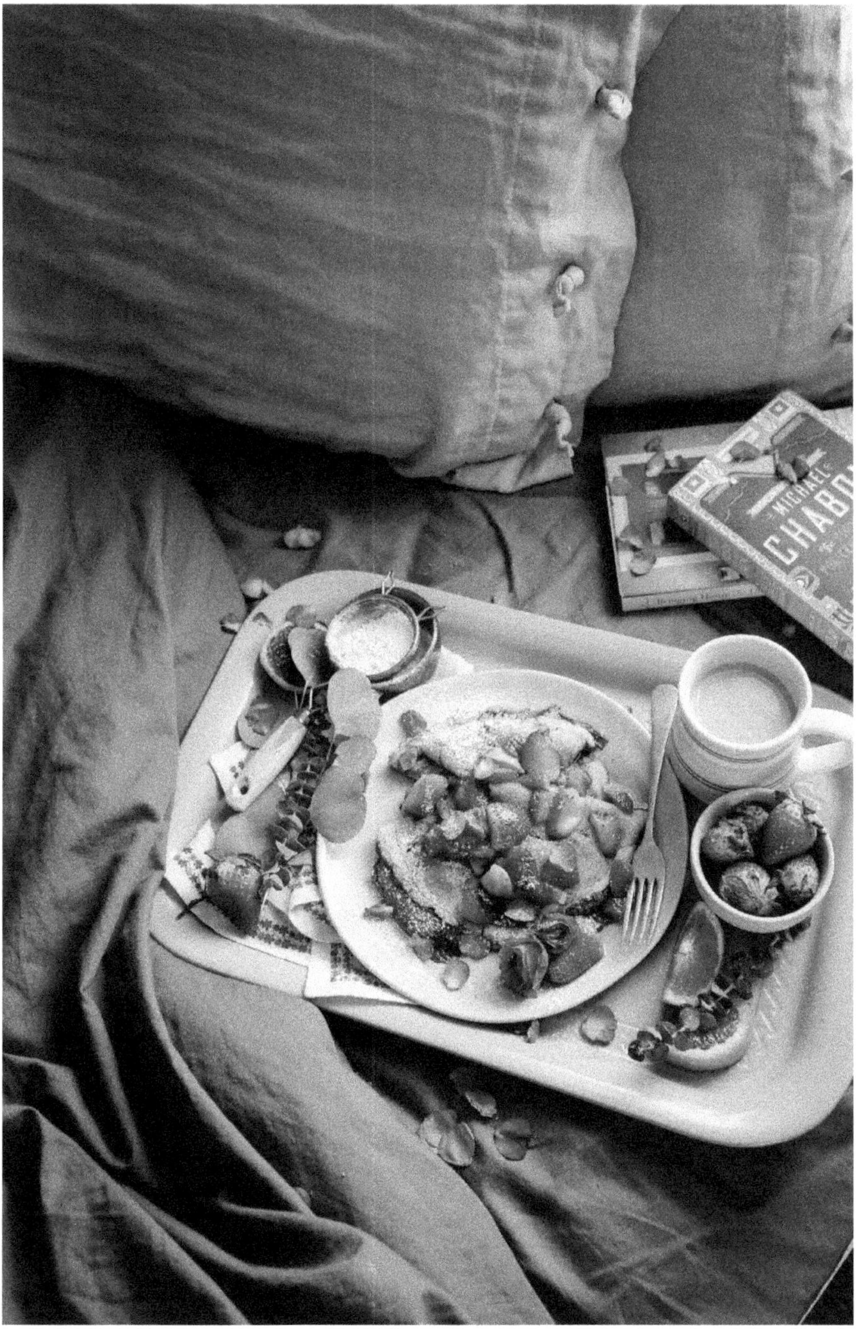

Recipes For Main Courses And Single Dishes

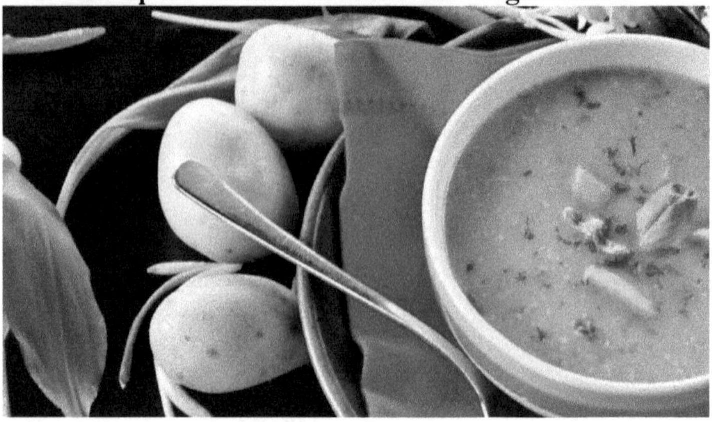

43 Spicy Cheesy Tofu Balls

Preparation Time: 30 minutesCooking Time: 15 minutes Servings: 4
Ingredients:

⅓ cup vegan mayonnaise

¼ cup pickled jalapenos1 pinch cayenne pepper

3 oz. grated vegan cheddar cheese1 tsp paprika powder
1 tbsp mustard powder

1 tbsp flax seed powder + 3 tbsp water2 ½ cup crumbled tofu
Salt and black pepper to taste

2 tbsp vegan butter, for fryingDirections:
For the spicy cheese:

In a bowl, mix all the ingredients for the spicy vegan cheese until well combined. Set aside.

In another medium bowl, combine the flax seed powder with water and allow soaking for 5 minutes.

Add the flax egg to the cheese mixture, the crumbled tofu, salt, and black pepper, and combine well. Use your hands to form large

meatballs out of the mix.

Melt the vegan butter in a large skillet over medium heat and fry thetofu balls until cooked and golden brown on all sides, 10 minutes.

Serve the tofu balls with your favorite mashes or in burgers.

44 Radish Chips

Preparation Time: 20 MinutesCooking Time: 10 Minutes Servings: 4
Ingredients:

10-15 Radishes, Large

Sea Salt & Black Pepper to TasteDirections:
Start by heating your oven to 375.

Slice your radishes thin, and then spread them out on a cookie sheetthat's been sprayed with cooking spray.

Mist the radishes with cooking spray, and then season with salt and pepper.

Bake for ten minutes, and then flip.

Bake for five to ten minutes more. They should be crispy.

Interesting Facts: Potatoes are a great starchy source of potassium and protein. They are pretty inexpensive if you are one that is watching their budget. Bonus: Very heart healthy!

45 Sautéed Pears

Preparation Time: 35 MinutesCooking Time: 30 Minutes Servings: 6
Ingredients:

2 Tablespoons Margarine (Or Vegan Butter)

¼ Teaspoon Cinnamon

¼ Teaspoon Nutmeg

6 Bosc Pears, Peeled & Quartered1 Tablespoon Lemon Juice
½ Cup Walnuts, Toasted & Chopped (Optional)Directions:
Melt your vegan butter in a skillet, and then add your spices. Cookfor a half a minute before adding in your pears.

Cook for fifteen minutes, and then stir in your lemon juice. Serve with walnuts if desired.
Interesting Facts: Cinnamon: This spice is an absolute powerhouse

and is considered one of the healthiest, beneficial spices on the plant. It's widely known for its medicinal properties. This spice is loaded with powerful antioxidants and is popular for its anti- inflammatory properties. It can reduce heart disease and lower bloodsugar levels.

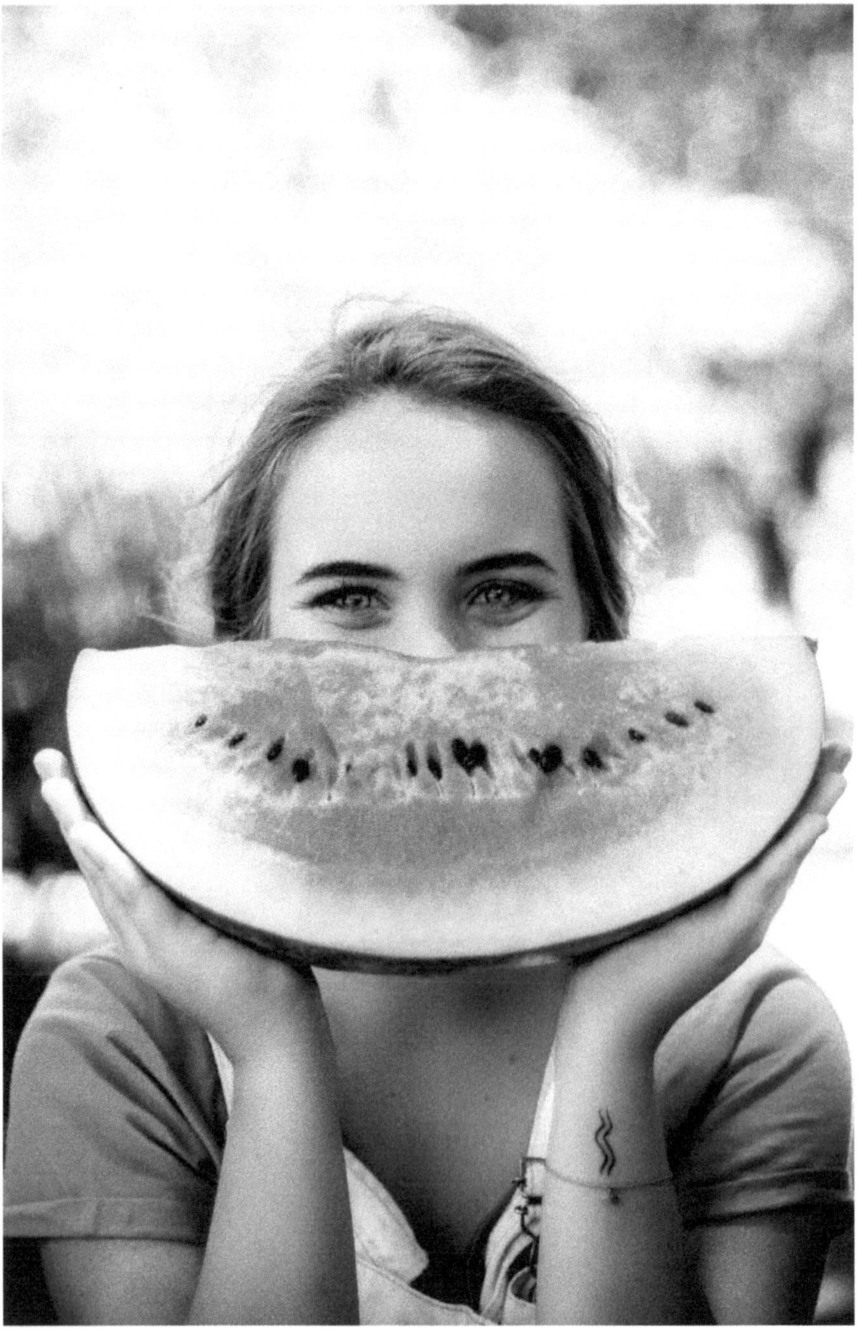

Nutrient-Packed Protein Salads

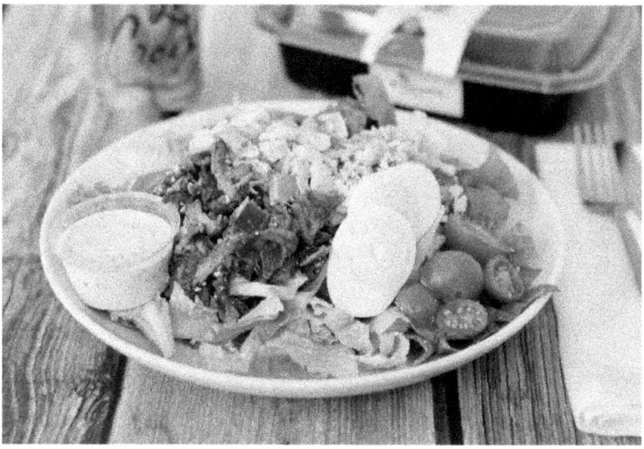

46 Red Cabbage Salad With Curried Seitan

Preparation time: 10 minsCooking time: 10 mins Ingredient:

1 Tbs. olive oil

1 8-oz. pkg. seitan, cut into bite-size strips 3 cloves garlic, minced (1 Tbs.)

¾ tsp. mild curry powder

6 cups shredded red cabbage (½ small head)

1 small cucumber, sliced into thin half-moons (¾ cup) 3 green onions, thinly sliced (½ cup)

⅓ cup prepared mango chutney

⅓ cup creamy natural peanut butter.

Directions:

To make Dressing: Blend chutney, peanut butter, and 1/3 cup water in blender until smooth. Set aside. To make Salad: Heat 2 tsp. oil in large skillet over medium heat. Add seitan, and season with salt, if desired. Sauté 5 to 7 minutes, or until browned. Add garlic andremaining 1 tsp. oil, and sauté 30 seconds. Sprinkle with curry powder, and sauté 2 minutes more. Remove from heat, and keep warm. Toss cabbage and cucumber with Dressing in large bowl. Top with warm seitan and green onions.

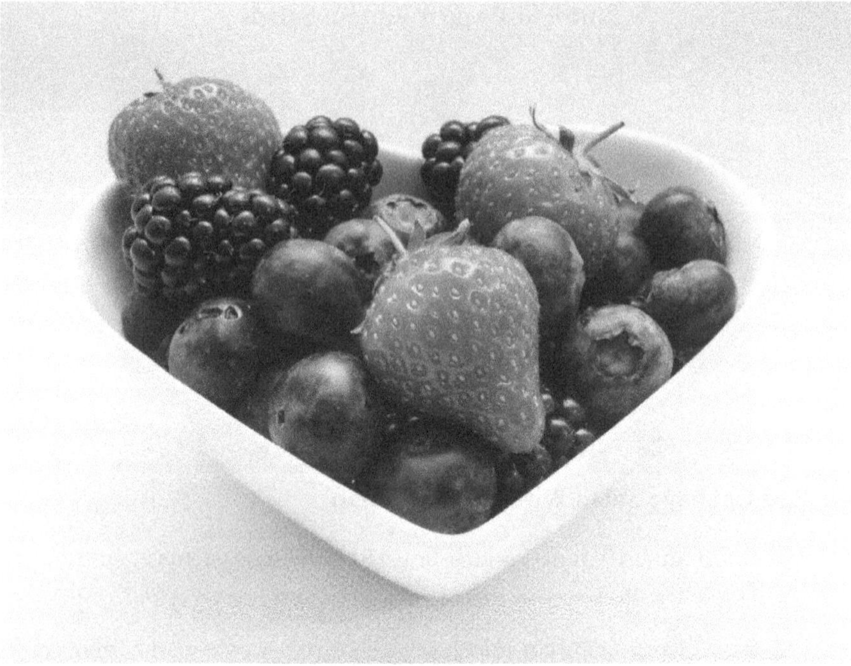

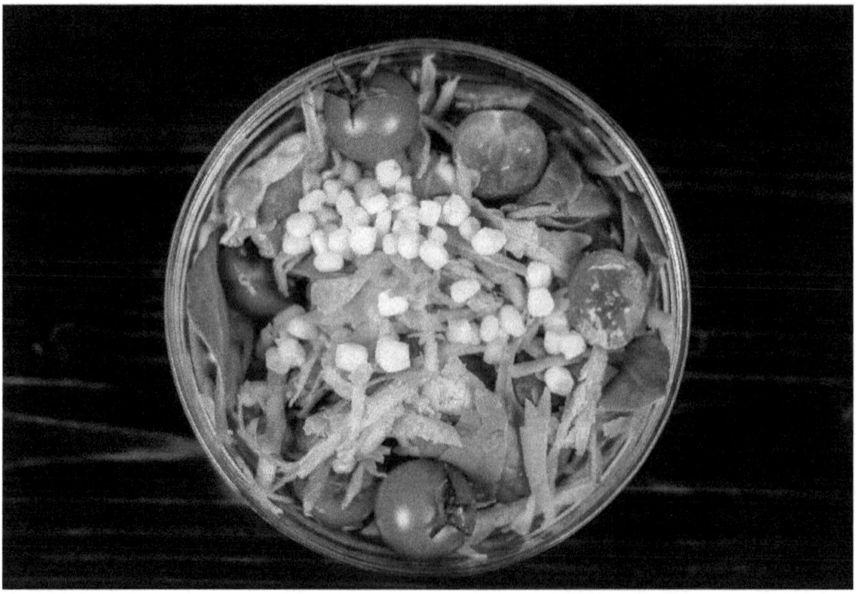

Flavour Boosters (Fish Glazes, Meat Rubs & Fish Rubs)

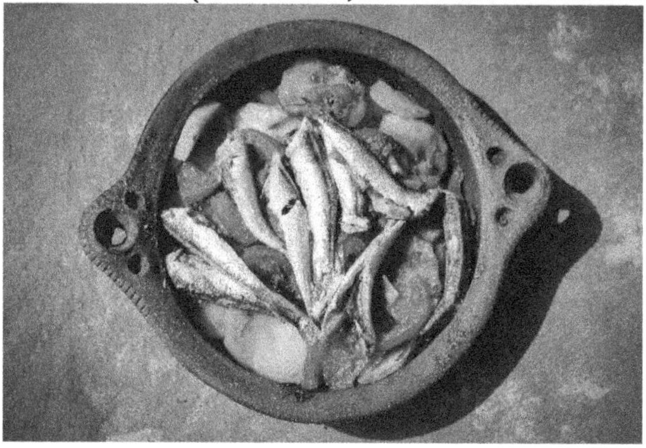

47 Rosemary Thyme Rub

This special rub recipe represents an interesting balance of spicyand sweet flavors to make truly mesmerizing meat meals.

A spiced combo of rosemary, thyme, and celery seeds never fails to produce delicious dishes with well-balanced flavors for the whole family.

Preparation Time: 5 min.

Cooking Time: 5 min. Servings: 1 cup/16 tbs.Ingredients:
Dried thyme - 1/4 cup

Dried crushed rosemary - 1/4 cupDry mustard - 2 tbs.
Ground black pepper - 4 tsp.Salt - 4 tsp.
Onion powder - 4 tsp.Ground cloves - 2 tsp.Celery seed - 2 tsp.
Cayenne- 1 tsp.Directions:
Mix in all mentioned rub ingredients in your mixing bowl to make the rosemary rub. Gently mix all ingredients using spatula or spoon to form an aromatic rub mixture.

Now, take your choice of meat cut and place it on a firm surface. Brush the freshly made rub on it; pat gently for the rub to stick onto the surface. Turn the meat cut and repeat to spice up its other side. Repeat with other meat cuts.

Let your meat cuts adequately season for more rich flavors for a few hours in your refrigerator. Take them out, as they are ready to be cooked or grilled!

48 Super Spiced Curry Rub

Your favorite meat cuts deserve a little jazzing up with this unique curry flavored rub. Paprika mixed with curry powder and cinnamon creates a perfect blend of spices. Be creative and add one or two of your favorite spices in it to come up with your own special version of spiced curry rub.

Preparation Time: 5 min.Cooking Time: 5 min.
Yield: 10 tbs.

Ingredients:

Ground ginger - 2 tbs.

Yellow curry powder - 3 tbs.Ground cinnamon - 2 tbs.
Salt - 1 tsp.

Mild paprika - 1 tbs. Ground cumin - 2 tbs. Ground allspice - 1 tsp.
Directions:
One by one, mix in all mentioned rub ingredients in your mixing bowl to make the curry rub. Gently mix all the ingredients using spatula or spoon to form an aromatic rub mixture.

Now, take your choice of meat cut and place it on a firm surface. Brush or rub the freshly made rub on it; pat gently for the rub to stick to the surface. Turn the meat cut and repeat to spice up its other side. Repeat with other meat cuts.

Let your meat cuts adequately season for more rich flavors for a few hours in your refrigerator. Take them out, as they are ready to be

cooked or grilled!

Sauce Recipes

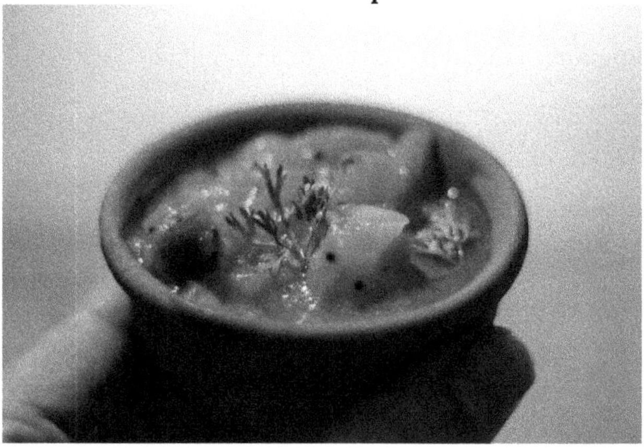

49 Vegan White Bean Gravy

Preparation time: 5 minutesCooking time: 5 minutes Servings: 2 1/5 cups
Ingredients:
1 cup of soy milk

1 cup vegetable broth

1 cup white beans, rinsed and drained

1 tablespoon nutritional yeast3 tablespoons tamari

1 teaspoon garlic granules, dried

2 teaspoons onion granules, dried2 tablespoons all-purpose flour
1 tablespoon combination thyme, oregano, dill, minced

1/4 teaspoon black pepper 1/4 teaspoon Himalayan saltDirections:
Add all ingredients except flour, herbs, and salt to a blender and blend on high speed until smooth.

Add this mixture to a pan placed over medium heat. Add salt, herbs,and flour, whisk all the time — Cook for 5 minutes.Serve and enjoy.

50 Tahini Maple Dressing

Preparation time: 5 minutesCooking time: 5 minutes Servings: 4 oz Ingredients

¼ cup tahini

1 ½ tablespoons maple syrup2 teaspoons lemon juice
¼ cup of water

1/8 teaspoon Himalayan pink saltDirections:

Add all the ingredients to a bowl, Stir well to combine, until well mixed.

Use as a dressing for the salad or other dishes. Store in a fridge.

Plant Based Diet for Women Over 50

Healthy Recipes to Lose Weight While Enjoy Tasty Food

Frank Smith

Breakfasts

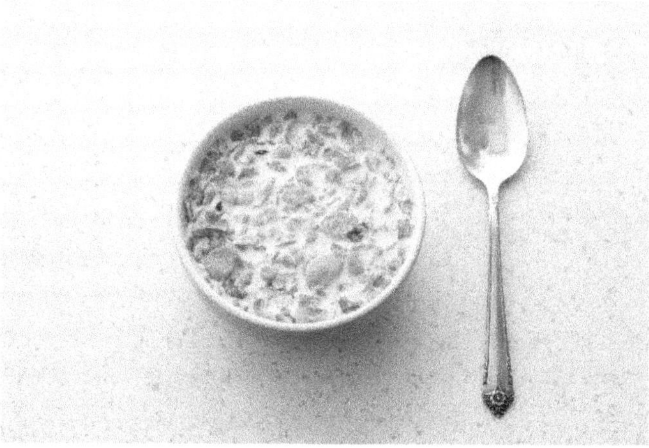

1 Orange Dream Creamsicle

Preparation time: 5 minutesCooking time: 5 minutes Servings: 2
Ingredients:

1 orange, peeled

¼ cup vegan yogurt2 tbsp. orange juice
¼ tsp vanilla extract4 ice cubes Directions:
In a blender, add orange, orange juice, vegan yogurt, vanilla extract and ice cubes. Blend all the ingredients well until smooth and well combined. Pour it into smoothie glasses and serve.

Nutrition: Calories 120 Carbohydrates 62 g Fats 6 g Protein 10g

2 Strawberry Limeade

Preparation time: 5 minutesCooking time: 5 minutes Servings: 6
Ingredients:

2 cup strawberries

1 cup sugar or as per taste7 cups of water
2 cup lemon juice

Sliced berries for garnishDirections:
Take a small bowl, add sugar and water and put in microwave until dissolved. Now take a blender and add strawberries and a cup of water and blend well. Combine the strawberries puree with the sugar dissolve water and mix. Pour lime juice and water if required. Stirwell and chill before serving. You can add berries on the top as garnishing.

Nutrition: Calories: 144, carbohydrates: 37g, sugar: 35g

3 Peanut Butter and Jelly Smoothie

Preparation time: 5 minutesCooking time: 5 minutes Servings: 2
Ingredients:

1 cup frozen raspberries 1 cup frozen strawberries
1 serving collagen peptides

1 tbsp. peanut butter

¾ cup almond milkDirections:
Take a blender. Add in raspberries, strawberries, peanut butter,

collagen peptide and almond milk. Blend all ingredients until well combined. Add almond milk as per the required consistency. Pour into smoothie serving glasses and top up with the peanut butter or anything of your choice for dressing.

Nutrition: Calories: 251, fat: 11.1g, carbohydrates: 27.5g, proteins: 15.7g

4 Banana Bread Breakfast Muffins

Preparation time: 40 mCooking time: 20 m Ingredients:
1/2 cup plus 2 tbs of whole oats 1/2 cup oats (processed into flour) 1/2 teaspoon baking powder

1 tablespoon vegan chocolate chips1/4 teaspoon cinnamon
1/2 cup of a mashed ripe banana (mash the banana and then measure it)

2 tablespoons pure maple syrup1/2 teaspoon vanilla extract Directions:
Preheat the cooker to 360 ° F and spray a muffin pan (3-4 holes) with a non-stick spray.

Add 1/2 cup oatmeal in a food processor and beat until it breaks and forms a thick consistency of flour.

In a large container, add all the dry ingredients except the chocolate chips and mix.

Crush and mash the uneven ripe banana, add the banana and the rest of the wet ingredients to the container with the dry ingredients and mix well.

Mix the chocolate chips. Put in 3-4 muffin holes and bake for 12 minutes.

Let cool 10 mins and serve immediately or store in an airtightcontainer for 1-2 days.

Nutrition: Per serving: Carbohydrates: 59g Calories: 347 Fat: 6gSodium: 2 mg Proteins: 15g Sugar: 1g

5 Breakfast Parfaits

Preparation: 15 minutesCooking: 0 minutes Servings: 2
Ingredients

One 14-ounce can coconut milk, refrigerated overnight1 cup granola ½ Cup walnuts

1 cup sliced strawberries or other seasonal berriesDirections
Pour off the canned coconut-milk liquid and retain the solids.

Intwoparfaitglasses, layerthecoconut-milksolids,granola, walnuts, and strawberries. Serve immediately.

6 Sweet Potato And Kale Hash

Preparation time: 10 minutesCooking time: 15 minutes Servings: 2
Ingredients

1 sweet potato

2 tablespoons olive oil

½ Onion, chopped

1 carrot, peeled and chopped2 garlic cloves, minced
½ Teaspoon dried thyme1 cup chopped kale
Sea salt

Freshly ground black pepperDirections
Prick the sweet potato with a fork and microwave on high until soft, about 5 minutes. Remove from the microwave and cut into ¼-inch cubes.

In a large nonstick sauté pan, heat the olive oil over medium-high heat. Add the onion and carrot and cook until softened, about 5 minutes. Add the garlic and thyme and cook until the garlic is fragrant, about 30 seconds.

Add the sweet potatoes and cook until the potatoes begin to brown, about 7 minutes. Add the kale and cook just until it wilts, 1 to 2 minutes. Season with salt and pepper. Serve immediately.

7 Delicious Oat Meal

Preparation time: 10 minutesCooking time: 6 hours Servings: 4
Ingredients:

3 cups water

3 cups almond milk

1 and ½ cups steel oats

4 dates, pitted and chopped

1 teaspoon cinnamon, ground2 tablespoons coconut sugar
½ Teaspoon ginger powder

A pinch of nutmeg, groundA pinch of cloves, ground 1 teaspoon vanilla extract Directions:
Put water and milk in your slow cooker and stir.

Add oats, dates, cinnamon, sugar, ginger, nutmeg, cloves and vanilla extract, stir, cover and cook on low for 6 hours.

Divide into bowls and serve for breakfast.Enjoy!
Nutrition: calories 120, fat 1, fiber 2, carbs 3, protein 5

8 Sweet Potato Toasts

Preparation time: 10 minutesCooking time: 10 minutes Servings: 2 Ingredients:

2 large sweet potatoes, sliced into ¼ inch thick slices1 tablespoon avocado oil
1 teaspoon salt

½ cup guacamole

½ cup tomatoes, slicedDirections:
Preheat your oven to 425 degrees F.

Cover a baking sheet with parchment paper.

Rub the potato slices with oil and salt and place them on a baking sheet.

Bake for 5 minutes in the oven, then flip and bake again for 5 minutes.

Top the baked slices with guacamole and tomatoes.Serve.
Nutrition: Calories134 Total Fat4.7gSaturatedFat.6g

Cholesterol 124mg Sodium 1 mg Total Carbs 54.1 g Fiber 7 g Sugar

3.3 g Protein 6.2 g

9 Tofu Scramble Tacos

Preparation time: 10 minutesCooking time: 10 minutes Servings: 04
Ingredients:

1 package tofu

¼ cup nutritional yeast

2 teaspoons garlic powder2 teaspoons cumin
2 teaspoons chili powder

½ teaspoon turmeric1 teaspoon salt
½ teaspoon pepper

1 tablespoon avocado oilWarm corn tortillas Directions:
In a pan, add avocado oil and tofu.

Sauté and crumble the tofu on medium heat.Stir in all the remaining spices and yeast.
Mix and cook for 2 minutes.Serve on tortillas.
Nutrition: Calories 387 Total Fat 6 g Saturated Fat 3.4 g Cholesterol 41 mg Sodium 154 mg Total Carbs 37.4 g Fiber 2.9 g Sugar 1.3 g Protein 6.6 g

10 Pumpkin Spice Bites

Preparation time: 10 minutesCooking time: 0 minutes Servings: 2
Ingredients:

½ cup pumpkin puree

½ cup almond butter

¼ cup maple syrup

1 teaspoon pumpkin pie spice1 ⅓ cup rolled oats
⅓ cup pumpkin seeds

⅓ cup raisins

2 tablespoons chia seedsDirections
In a sealable container, add everything and mix well.Seal the container and refrigerate overnight.
Roll the mixture into small balls.Serve.
Nutrition:Calories212TotalFat11.8gSaturatedFat2.2 g

Cholesterol 23mg Sodium 321 mg Total Carbs 14.6 g Fibers 4.4 g Sugar 8 g Protein 7.3g

11 Lemon Spelt Scones

Preparation time: 10 minutesCooking time: 18 minutes Servings: 6
Ingredients:

1¾ cups spelt flour1¼ cup whole spelt
⅔ cup coconut sugar

2 teaspoons baking powder

½ teaspoon salt

3 tablespoons lemon zest

½ cup coconut oil

1 cup coconut cream

2 tablespoons almond milk2 cups frozen raspberries Directions
Preheat your oven to 425 degrees F.

Whisk dry ingredients in a stand mixer using whisk attachment.

Freeze the dry mixture for 10 minutes then place it back on the mixer.

Using the paddle attachment, stir in coconut oil, coconut cream, and almond milk then beat until smooth.

Fold in frozen raspberries and mix again, divide the dough into two parts.

Spread each part into a thick disk and cut each into 6 wedges of equal size.

Line a suitable baking sheet with parchment paper and place the wedges on the tray.

Bake for 18 minutes then serve.

Nutrition: Calories 119 Total Fat 14 g Saturated Fat 2 g Cholesterol 65 mg Sodium 269 mg Total Carbs 19 g Fiber 4 g Sugar 6 g Protein 5g

12 Veggie Breakfast Scramble

Preparation time: 10 minutesCooking time: 14 minutes Servings: 06
Ingredients:

1 cup yellow onions, chopped 1 cup red bell peppers, diced 1½ cups zucchini, sliced
3 cups cauliflower florets

1 tablespoon garlic, minced1 tablespoon tamari
2 tablespoons vegetable broth

2 tablespoons nutritional yeast

1 (15 ounce) can chickpeas, drained2 cups baby spinach, chopped Spice Mix:
1 teaspoon onion powder

1 teaspoon garlic powder

1 teaspoon dried minced onions

¾ teaspoon dried ground mustard powder1 teaspoon dried thyme leaves
1 teaspoon smoked paprika

¼ teaspoon turmeric

¾ teaspoon salt

¼ teaspoon black pepperDirections
In a suitable pan, add cooking oil and all the vegetables.

Cook while stirring for 7 minutes on medium heat.Toss in the chickpeas and all the spices.
Continue sautéing for another 7 minutes.

Serve warm.

Nutrition:Calories231TotalFat20.1gSaturatedFat2.4g Cholesterol 110 mg Sodium 941 mg Total Carbs 20.1 g Fiber 0.9 g
Sugar 1.4 g Protein 4.6 g

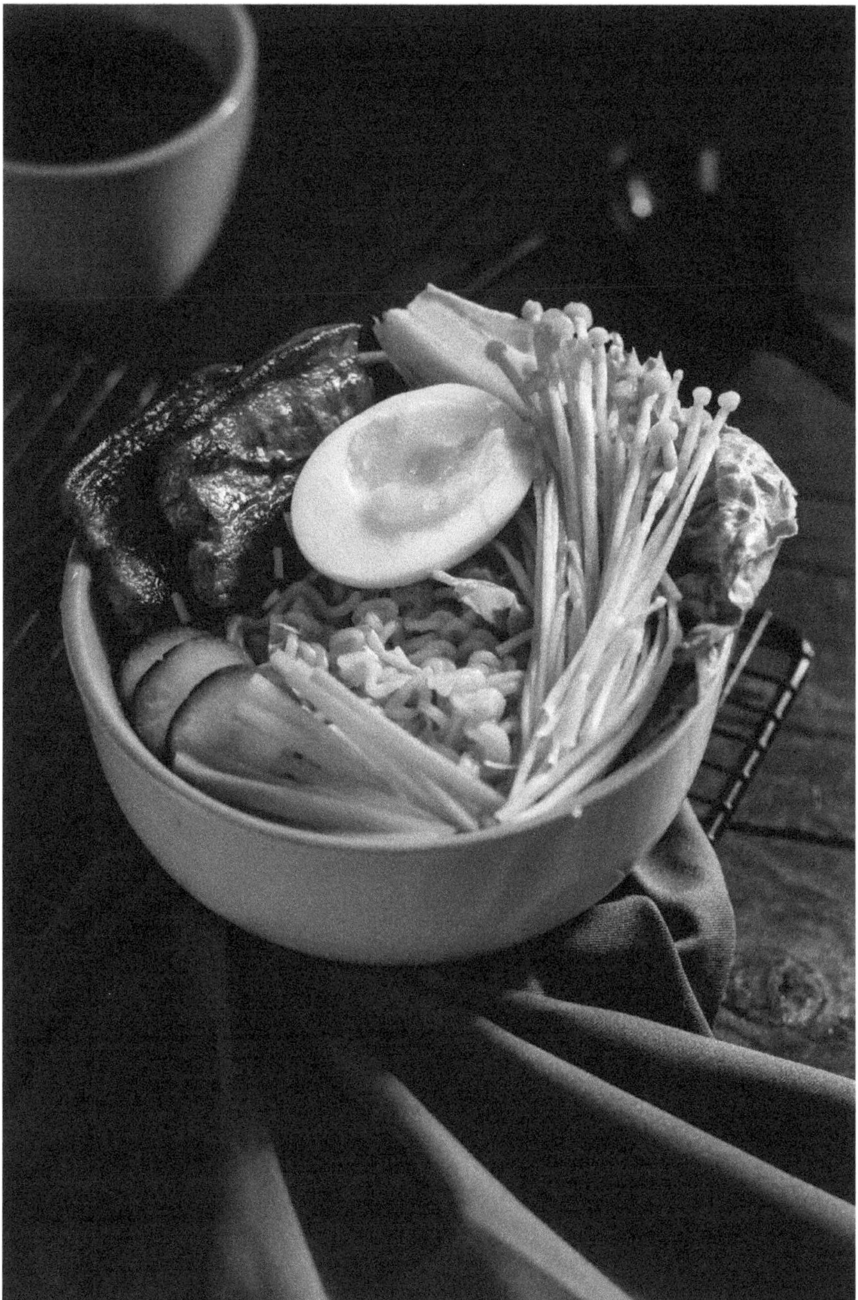

Soups, Salads, and Sides

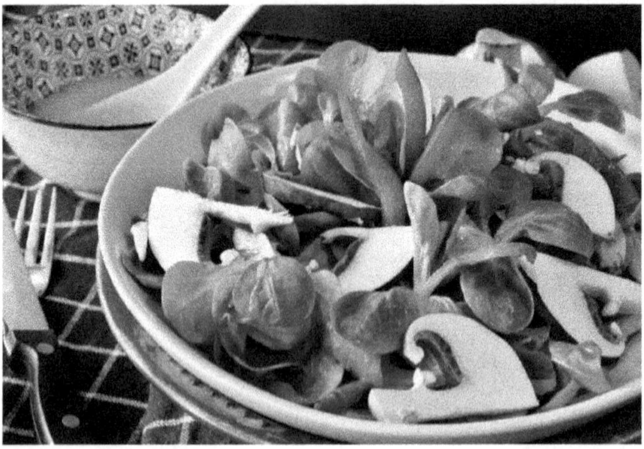

13 Tamari Toasted Almonds

Preparation time: 2 minutes Cooking time: 8 minutes Servings: ½ cup Ingredients:
½ cup raw almonds, or sunflower seeds2 tablespoons tamari, or soy sauce
1 teaspoon toasted sesame oil

Directions:

Preparing the ingredients.

Heat a dry skillet to medium-high heat, then add the almonds, stirringvery frequently to keep them from burning. Once the almonds are toasted, 7 to 8 minutes for almonds, or 3 to 4 minutes for sunflower seeds, pour the tamari and sesame oil into the hot skillet and stir to coat.

You can turn off the heat, and as the almonds cool the tamari mixturewill stick to and dry on the nuts.

Nutrition: calories: 89; total fat: 8g; carbs: 3g; fiber: 2g; protein: 4g

14 Nourishing Whole-Grain Porridge

Preparation time: 2 hours and 10 minutesCooking time: 2 hours
Servings: 4

Ingredients:

3/4 cup of steel-cut oats, rinsed and soaked overnight3/4 cup of whole barley, rinsed and soaked overnight 1/2 cup of cornmeal
1 teaspoon of salt

3 tablespoons of brown sugar

1 cinnamon stick, about 3 inches long

1 teaspoon of vanilla extract, unsweetened4 1/2 cups of water
Directions:

Using a 6-quarts slow cooker, place all the ingredients and stirproperly.

Cover it with the lid, plug in the slow cooker and let it cook for 2 hours or until grains get soft, while stirring halfway through.

Serve the porridge with fruits.

Nutrition:Calories:129Cal,arbohydrates:22g,Protein:5g,Fats:2g, Fiber:4g.

15 Pungent Mushroom Barley Risotto

Preparation time: 3 hours and 30 minutes Cooking time: 3 hours and 9 minutes Servings: 4
Ingredients:

1 1/2 cups of hulled barley, rinsed and soaked overnight 8 ounces of carrots, peeled and chopped
1 pound of mushrooms, sliced

1 large white onion, peeled and chopped3/4 teaspoon of salt
1/2 teaspoon of ground black pepper4 sprigs thyme
1/4 cup of chopped parsley

2/3 cup of grated vegan Parmesan cheese 1 tablespoon of apple cider vinegar
2 tablespoons of olive oil

1 1/2 cups of vegetable brothDirections:
Place a large non-stick skillet pan over a medium-high heat, add theoil and let it heat until it gets hot.

Add the onion along with 1/4 teaspoon of each the salt and black pepper.

Cook it for 5 minutes or until it turns golden brown.

Then add the mushrooms and continue cooking for 2 minutes. Add the barley, thyme and cook for another 2 minutes.
Transfer this mixture to a 6-quarts slow cooker and add the carrots,

1/4 teaspoon of salt, and the vegetable broth. Stir properly and cover it with the lid.
Plug in the slow cooker, let it cook for 3 hours at the high heat setting

or until the grains absorb all the cooking liquid and the vegetablesget soft.

Remove the thyme sprigs, pour in the remaining ingredients exceptfor parsley and stir properly.

Pour in the warm water and stir properly until the risotto reaches your desired state.

Add the seasoning, then garnish it with parsley and serve.

Nutrition:alories:321Cal,Carbohydrates:48g,Protein:12g, Fats:10g,

Fiber:11g.

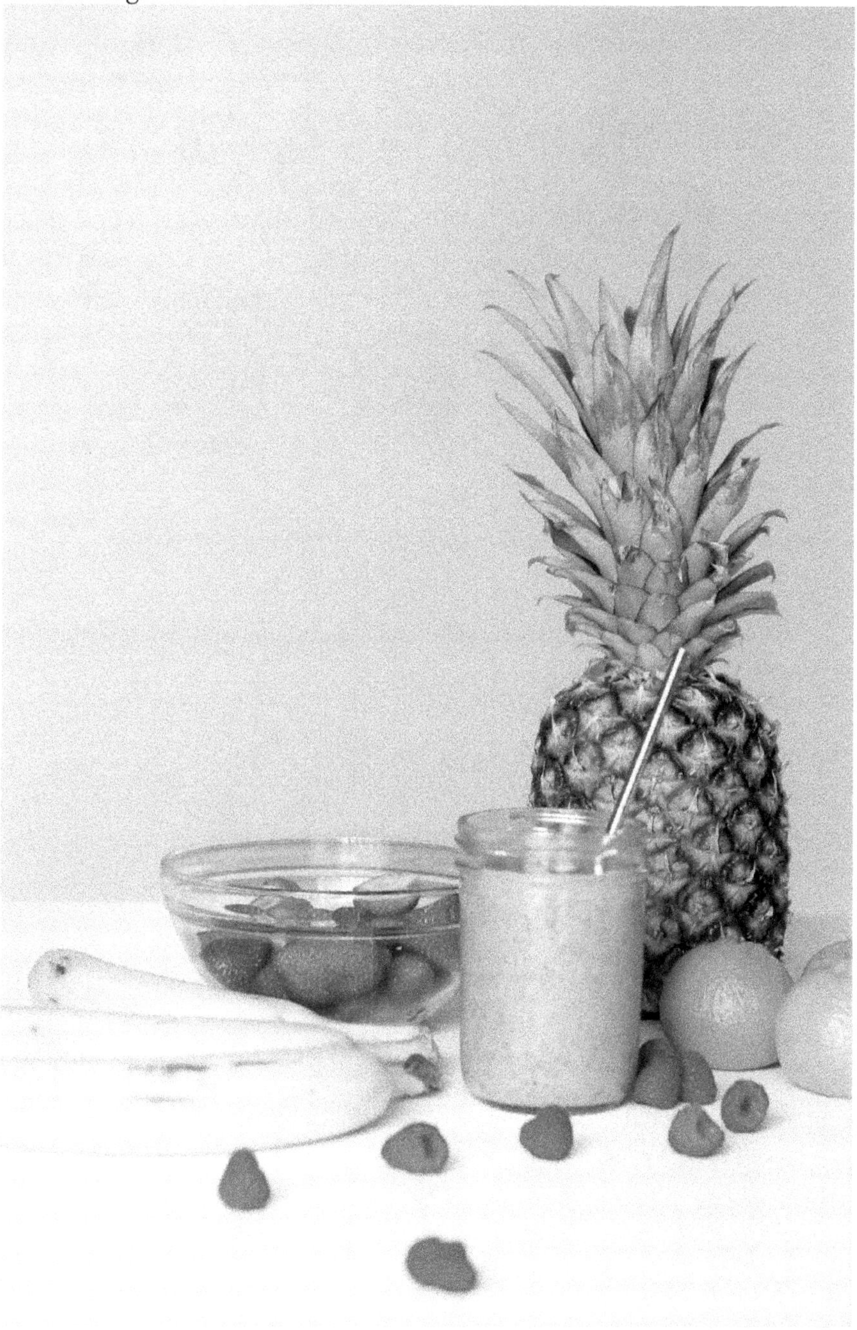

Entrées

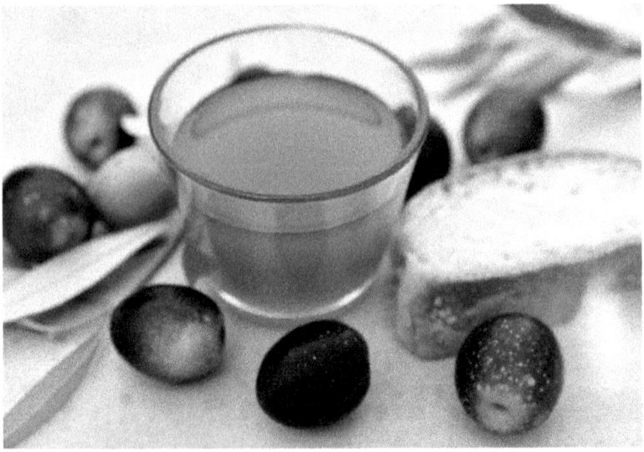

16 Oven Baked Sesame Fries

Preparation time: 30 minutesCooking time: 30 minutes Servings: 4
Ingredients:

1 pound Yukon Gold potatoes, skins on and cut into wedges2 tablespoons sesame seeds
1 tablespoon potato starch

1 tablespoon sesame oilSalt to taste
Black pepper to tasteDirections:
Preheat the oven to 425 degrees, Fahrenheit and cover a baking sheet or two with parchment paper.

Cut the potatoes and place in a large bowl.

Add the sesame seeds, potato starch, sesame oil, salt and pepper.

Toss with your hands and make sure all the wedges are coated. Addmore sesame seeds or oil if needed.

Spread the potato wedges on the baking sheets with some room between each wedge.

Bake for 15 minutes, flip the wedges over and then return them tothe oven for 10 to 15 more minutes, until they look golden and crispy.

17 Pumpkin Orange Spice Hummus

Preparation: 30 minutesCooking: 30 minutes Servings: 3
Ingredients:

1 cup canned, unsweetened pumpkin puree

1 16-ounce can garbanzo beans, rinsed and drained 1 tablespoon apple cider vinegar
1 tablespoon maple syrup

¼ cup tahini

1 tablespoon fresh orange juice

½ teaspoon orange zest and additional zest for garnish

⅛ teaspoon ground cinnamon

⅛ teaspoon ground ginger ⅛ teaspoon ground nutmeg

¼ teaspoon saltDirections:
Pour the pumpkin puree and garbanzo beans into a food processor and pulse to break up.

Add the vinegar, syrup, tahini, orange juice and orange zest pulse a few times.

Add the cinnamon, ginger, nutmeg and salt and process until smooth and creamy.

Serve in a bowl sprinkled with more orange zest with wheat crackers alongside.

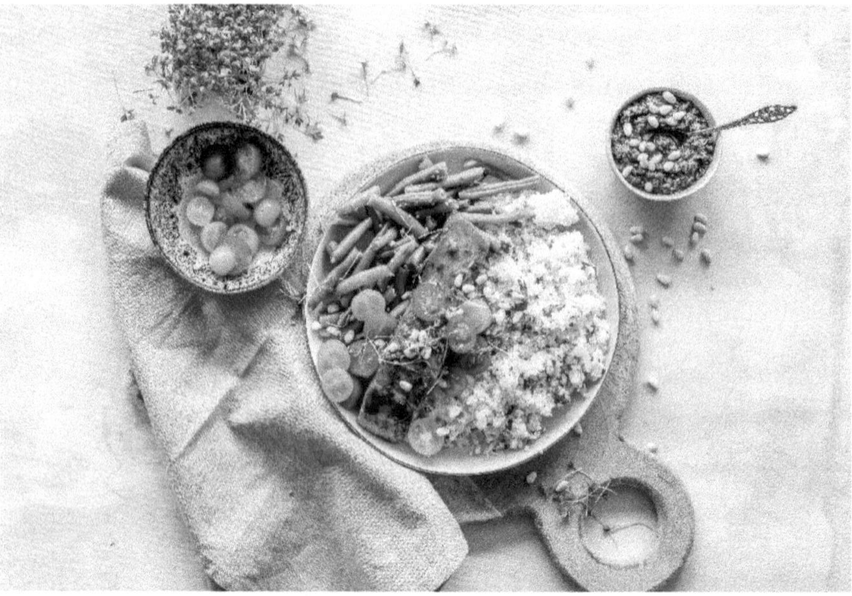

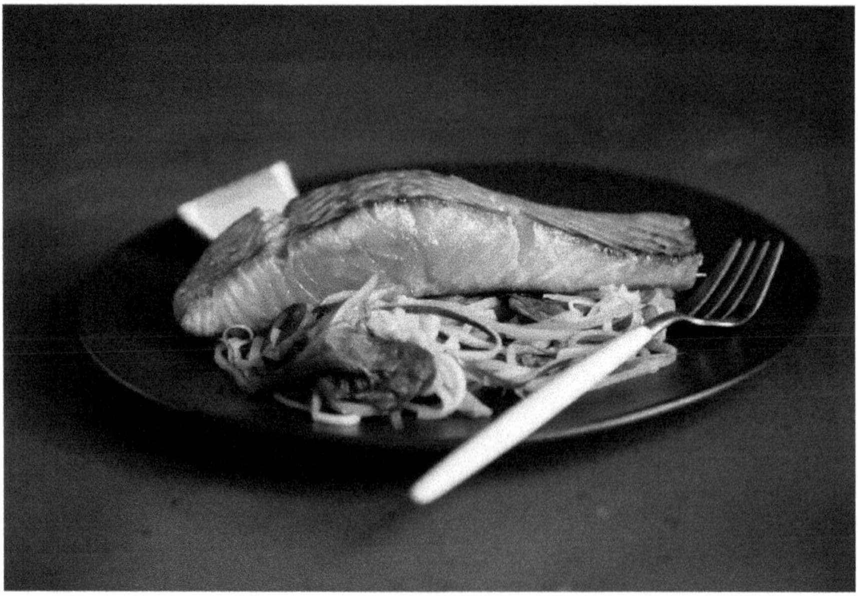

Smoothies and Beverages

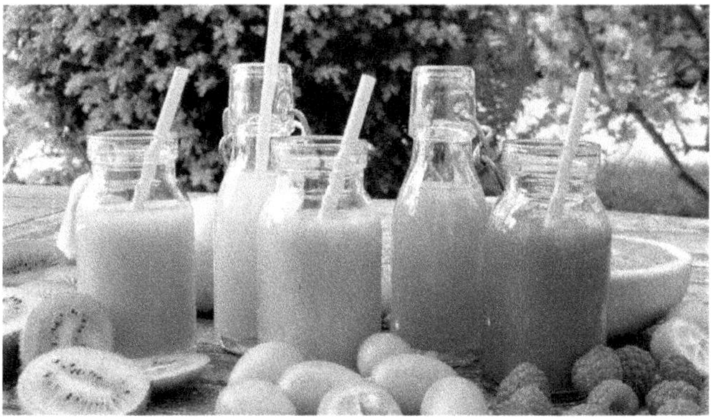

18 Cantaloupe Smoothie Bowl

Preparation Time: 5 MinutesCooking Time: 0 minutes Serves: 2
Calories: 135

Protein: 3 Grams

Fat: 1 Gram

Carbs: 32 GramsIngredients:
¾ Cup carrot Juice

4 Cps Cantaloupe, Frozen & CubedMellon Balls or Berries to Serve Pinch Sea Salt
Directions:

Blend everything together until smooth.

19 Berry & Cauliflower Smoothie

Preparation: 10 MinutesCooking: 0 minutes Serves: 2
Calories: 149 Protein: 3 Grams Fat: 3 Grams

Carbs: 29 GramsIngredients:
1 Cup Riced Cauliflower, Frozen

1 Cup Banana, Sliced & Frozen

½ Cup Mixed Berries, Frozen

2 Cups Almond Milk, Unsweetened

2 Teaspoons Maple syrup, Pure & OptionalDirections:
Blend until mixed well.

20 Green Mango Smoothie

Preparation Time: 5 MinutesCooking Time: 0 minutes Serves: 1
Calories: 417

Protein: 7.2 Grams

Fat: 2.8 Grams

Carbs: 102.8 GramsIngredients:
2 Cups Spinach

1-2 Cups Coconut Water

2 Mangos, Ripe, Peeled & DicedDirections:
Blend everything together until smooth.

21 Apricot Tarte Tatin

Preparation Time: 30 minutes + 1 hour chillingServings: 4
The fruit variety is the best overall, but it also goes well with apricots

– happiness on a table.Ingredients
For the piecrust:

4 tbsp flax seed powder + 12 tbsp water

¼ cup almond flour + extra for dusting3 tbsp whole-wheat flour
½ tsp salt

¼ cup plant butter, cold and crumbled3 tbsp pure maple syrup
1 ½ tsp vanilla extractFor the filling:
4 tbsp melted plant butter + more for brushing

3 tsp pure maple syrup1 tsp vanilla extract
1 lemon, juiced

12 apricots, halved and pitted

½ cup coconut cream

3 to 4 fresh basil leaves to garnishDirections

Preheat the oven to 350 F and grease a large pie pan with cooking spray.

In a medium bowl, mix the flax seed powder with water and allow thickening for 5 minutes.

In a large bowl, combine the flours and salt. Add the plant butter and using an electric hand mixer, whisk until crumbly. Pour in the flax egg, maple syrup, vanilla, and mix until smooth dough forms. Flatten the dough on a flat surface, cover with plastic wrap, and refrigerate for 1 hour.

After, lightly dust a working surface with almond flour, remove the dough onto the surface, and using a rolling pin, flatten the dough into a 1-inch diameter circle. Set aside.

In a large bowl, mix the plant butter, maple syrup, vanilla, and lemon juice. Add the apricots to the mixture and coat well.

Arrange the apricots (open side down) in the pie pan and lay the dough on top. Press to fit and cut off the dough hanging on the edges. Brush the top with more plant butter and bake in the oven for 35 to 40 minutes or until golden brown, and puffed up.

Remove the pie pan from the oven, allow cooling for 5 minutes, and run a butter knife around the edges of the pastry. Invert the dessert onto a large plate, spread the coconut cream on top, and garnish with the basil leaves. Slice and serve.

Nutritional info per serving

Calories 484 | Fats 33.8g| Carbs 46.4g | Protein 2.8g

22 Chocolate & Pistachio Popsicles

Preparation Time: 5 minutes + 3 hours chilling

Servings: 4

A popsicle is one of those wonders full of endless possibilities thatare creative and mouth-watering.

Ingredients

½ cup unsweetened chocolate chips, melted1 ½ cups oat milk
1 tbsp unsweetened cocoa powder

3 tbsp pure date syrup1 tsp vanilla extract
A handful pistachios, choppedDirections
In a blender, add chocolate, oat milk, cocoa powder, date syrup, vanilla, pistachios, and process until smooth. Divide the mixture into popsicle molds and freeze for 3 hours.

Dip the popsicle molds in warm water to loosen the popsicles and pull out the popsicles.

Nutritional info per serving

Calories 315 | Fats 17.8g| Carbs 34.9g | Protein 11.9g

23 Strawberry Cupcakes With Cashew Cheese Frosting

Preparation Time: 35 minutes + 30 minutes chillingServings: 4

To make this lovely pink ganache, you just need three basic ingredients. With freshly strawberry puree, it takes on a buttery flavor.

Ingredients

For the cupcakes:

2 cups whole-wheat flour

¼ cup cornstarch

2 ½ tsp baking powder

1 ½ cups pure date sugar

½ tsp salt

¾ cup unsalted plant butter, room temperature3 tsp vanilla extract
1 cup strawberries, pureed

1 cup oat milk, room temperatureFor the frosting:
¾ cup cashew cream

2 tbsp coconut oil, melted3 tbsp pure maple syrup 1 tsp vanilla extract
1 tsp freshly squeezed lemon juice

¼ tsp salt

2-4 tbsp water as needed for blendingDirections

Preheat the oven to 350 F and line a 12-holed muffin tray with cupcake liners. Set aside.

In a large bowl, mix the flour, cornstarch, baking powder, date sugar,and salt.

Using an electric mixer, whisk in the plant butter, vanilla extract, strawberries, and oat milk until well combined.

Divide the mixture into the muffin cups two-thirds way up and bake inthe oven for 20 to 25 minutes or until golden brown on top and a toothpick inserted comes out clean. Remove the cupcakes and allow cooling while you make the frosting.

In a blender, add the cashew cream, coconut oil, maple syrup, vanilla, lemon juice, and salt. Process until smooth. If the mixture is too thick, add some water to lighten the consistency a little. Pour the frosting into medium and chill for 30 minutes.

Transfer the mixture into a piping bag and swirl mounds of the frosting onto the cupcakes. Serve immediately.

Nutritional info per serving

Calories 853 | Fats 42g| Carbs 112.8g | Protein 14.3g

24 Nut Stuffed Sweet Apples

Preparation Time: 35 minutesServings: 4

This nut Stuffed Baked Apples are a buzz-friendly sliding dessert, orsay, one or two weekend desserts snack.

Ingredients

4 gala apples

3 tbsp pure maple syrup4 tbsp almond flour
6 tbsp pure date sugar

6 tbsp plant butter, cold and cubed1 cup chopped mixed nuts

Directions

Preheat the oven the 400 F.

Slice off the top of the apples and use a melon baller or spoon to scoop out the cores of the apples. In a bowl, mix the maple syrup, almond flour, date sugar, butter, and nuts.

Spoon the mixture into the apples and then bake in the oven for 25 minutes or until the nuts are golden brown on top and the apples soft. Remove the apples from the oven, allow cooling, and serve.

Nutritional info per serving

Calories 581 | Fats 43.6g| Carbs 52.1g | Protein 3.6g

Snacks and Desserts

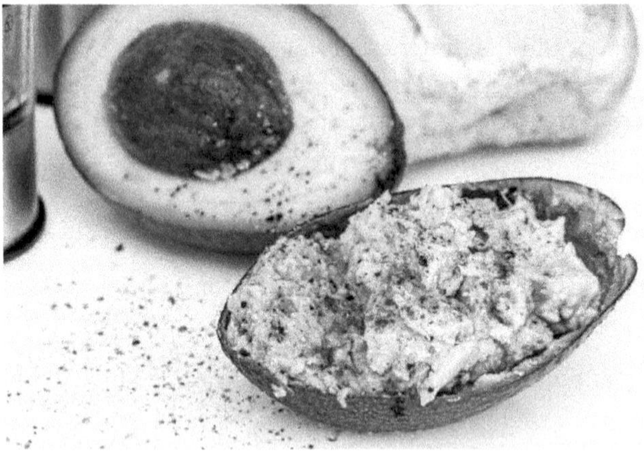

25 Curried Tofu "Egg Salad" Pitas

Preparation Time: 15 minutes Cooking time: 0 minutes Servings: 4 sandwiches Ingredients
1 pound extra-firm tofu, drained and patted dry

½ cup vegan mayonnaise, homemade or store-bought

¼ cup chopped mango chutney, homemade or store-bought 2 teaspoons Dijon mustard
1 tablespoon hot or mild curry powder

1 teaspoon salt

⅛ teaspoon ground cayenne

¾ cup shredded carrots2 celery ribs, minced
¼ cup minced red onion

8 small Boston or other soft lettuce leaves 4 (7-inch) whole wheat pita breads, halvedDirections
Crumble the tofu and place it in a large bowl. Add the mayonnaise, chutney, mustard, curry powder, salt, and cayenne, and stir well until thoroughly mixed.

Add the carrots, celery, and onion and stir to combine. Refrigeratefor 30 minutes to allow the flavors to blend.

Tuck a lettuce leaf inside each pita pocket, spoon some tofu mixtureon top of the lettuce, and serve.

26 Garden Salad Wraps

Preparation Time: 15 minutesCooking time: 10 minutes Servings: 4 wraps
Ingredients
6 tablespoons olive oil

1 pound extra-firm tofu, drained, patted dry, and cut into ½-inchstrips

1 tablespoon soy sauce

¼ cup apple cider vinegar

1 teaspoon yellow or spicy brown mustard

½ teaspoon salt

¼ teaspoon freshly ground black pepper3 cups shredded romaine lettuce
3 ripe Roma tomatoes, finely chopped

1 large carrot, shredded

1 medium English cucumber, peeled and chopped

⅓ cup minced red onion

¼ cup sliced pitted green olives

4 (10-inch) whole-grain flour tortillas or lavash flatbreadDirections
In a large skillet, heat 2 tablespoons of the oil over medium heat. Add the tofu and cook until golden brown, about 10 minutes. Sprinkle with soy sauce and set aside to cool.

In a small bowl, combine the vinegar, mustard, salt, and pepper with the remaining 4 tablespoons oil, stirring to blend well. Set aside.

In a large bowl, combine the lettuce, tomatoes, carrot, cucumber, onion, and olives. Pour on the dressing and toss to coat.

To assemble wraps, place 1 tortilla on a work surface and spread with about one-quarter of the salad. Place a few strips of tofu on the tortilla and roll up tightly. Slice in half 76.

27 Tamari Toasted Almonds

Preparation Time: 2 minutesCooking time: 8 minutes Servings: ½ cup
Ingredients

½ cup raw almonds, or sunflower seeds2 tablespoons tamari, or soy sauce
1 teaspoon toasted sesame oil

Directions

Preparing the Ingredients.

Heat a dry skillet to medium-high heat, then add the almonds, stirringvery frequently to keep them from burning. Once the almonds are toasted, 7 to 8 minutes for almonds, or 3 to 4 minutes for sunflower seeds, pour the tamari and sesame oil into the hot skillet and stir to coat.

You can turn off the heat, and as the almonds cool the tamari mixturewill stick to and dry on the nuts.

Per Serving (1 tablespoon) Calories: 89; Total fat: 8g; Carbs: 3g; Fiber: 2g; Protein: 4g

28 Protein-Rich Pumpkin Bowl

Preparation: 10 minutesCooking: 0 minutes Servings: 2
Ingredients

1 1/2 upsalmondmilk(moreorlessdependingondesiredconsistency)

1 cup pumpkin puree canned, with salt1/2 cup chopped walnuts
1 scoop vegan soy protein powder1 tsp pure vanilla extract
A handful of cacao nibsDirections:
Add all ingredients in a blender apart from the cacao nibs. Blend until smooth.Serve in bowls and sprinkle with cacao nibs.

29 Savory Red Potato-Garlic Balls

Preparation time: 40 minutesCooking time: 25 minutes Servings: 4
Ingredients

1 1/2 lbs of red potatoes

3 cloves of garlic finely chopped

1 Tbsp of fresh finely chopped parsley1/4 tsp ground turmeric
Salt and ground pepper to taste

Directions:

Rinse potatoes and place unpeeled into a large pot. Pour water to cover potatoes and bring to boil.
Cook for about 20 to 25 minutes on medium heat.

Rinse potatoes and let them cool down.

Peel potatoes and mash them; add finely chopped garlic, and thesalt and pepper.

Form the potato mixture into small balls.

Sprinkle with chopped parsley and refrigerate for several hours.Serve.

30 Spicy Smooth Red Lentil Dip

Preparation time: 35 minutesCooking time: 20 minutes Servings: 4
Ingredients

1 cup red lentils1 bay leaf
Sea salt to taste

2 garlic clove, finely chopped

2 Tbsp chopped cilantro leaves1 Tbsp tomato paste
Lemon juice from 2 lemons, freshly squeezed

2 tsp ground cumin

4 Tbsp extra-virgin olive oilDirections:
Rinse lentils and drain.

Combine lentils and bay leaf in a medium saucepan.

Pour enough water to cover lentils completely, and bring to boil.

Cover tightly, reduce heat to medium, and simmer for about 20minutes.

Season salt to taste, and stir well. Note: Always season with the saltafter cooking – if salt is added before, the lentils will become tough.

Drain the lentils in a colander. Discard the bay leaf and let the lentilscool for 10 minutes.

Transfer the lentils to a food processor and add all remaining ingredients.

Pulse until all ingredients combined well. Taste and adjust seasonings if needed.
Transfer a lentil dip into a glass container and refrigerate at least 2

hours before serving.

31 Apple Cinnamon Crisps

Preparation Time: 2 HoursCooking Time: 2 Hours Servings: 2
Ingredients:

Cinnamon (1 t.)

Apple (1, Sliced)Directions:
This recipe is simple and delicious! You can start off by turning the

oven to 200. As this warms up, you'll want to prep a baking sheet with some parchment paper.

With the baking sheet set, layout your apple slices across it evenly and sprinkle with the cinnamon. Once this is done, pop the dish into the oven for two hours.

Remove from oven, allow to cool, and enjoy.

Nutrition: Calories: 50 Proteins: 5g Carbs: 14g Fats: 1g

32 Steamed Broccoli with Sesame

Preparation: 15 minutesCooking: 5 minutes Servings: 2
Ingredients

1 1/2 lb fresh broccoli florets1/2 cup sesame oil
4 Tbsp sesame seedsSalt and ground pepper to tasteDirections:
Place broccoli florets in a steamer basket above boiling water. Cover and steam for about 4 to 5 minutes.
Remove from steam and place broccoli in serving the dish.Season with the salt and pepper, and drizzle with sesame oil; toss tocoat.

Sprinkle with sesame seeds and serve immediately.

33 Vegan Eggplant Patties

Preparation time: 30 minutesCooking time: 15 minutes Servings: 6
Ingredients

2 big eggplants

1 onion finely diced

1 Tbsp smashed garlic cloves 1 bunch raw parsley, chopped 1/2 cup almond meal

4 Tbsp Kalamata olives, pitted and sliced1 Tbsp baking soda

Salt and ground pepper to taste Olive oil or avocado oil, for frying

Directions

Peel off eggplants, rinse, and cut in half.

Sauté eggplant cubes in a non-stick skillet - occasionally stirring - about 10 minutes.

Transfer to a large bowl and mash with an immersion blender.Add eggplant puree into a bowl and add in all remaining ingredients(except oil).

Knead a mixture using your hands until the dough is smooth, sticky,and easy to shape.Shape mixture into 6 patties.Heat the olive oil in a frying skillet on medium-high heat.Fry patties for about 3 to 4 minutes per side.

Remove patties on a platter lined with kitchen paper towel to drain.Serve warm.

34 Vegan Breakfast Sandwich

Preparation Time: 10minutesCooking Time: 10 minutes Servings: 3
Ingredients

1 tsp. coconut oil6 slices of bread 1 14 oz container
1-2 tsp. veganextra firm tofumayo
1 tsp. turmeric 1 cup of greens1/2 tsp. garlic
1-2 medium powder tomatoes 1/2 tsp. Kala
6 pickle slicesNamak (blackFresh crackedsalt)

pepper

3 melty vegancheese slicesDirections:
Season one facet of the tofu with salt, garlic powder, break uppepper, and turmeric. I just 15 sprinkled it out of the flavor bins. You will season the second side within the field when it is a perfect possibility to flip them.

In a medium skillet, warmth oil over medium warmth and notice the tofu cuts organized aspect down on the dish. While the bottom facet is cooking, season the pinnacle side. Let the tofu cook dinner for three to 5 minutes, till marginally darker and clean. Presently turn the cuts over and fry the alternative aspect for 3-5 minutes. Presently's a respectable time to pop the bread in the toaster, on every occasion liked.

To liquefy the cheddar, on a preparing sheet, place 2 cuts of tofu onenext to the opposite, with a reduce of cheddar over every set. Put it within the broiler on prepare dinner for 1-three minutes, until the cheddar is dissolved. You can likewise utilize a toaster broiler.

Spread mayo on the two aspects of the bread.

Spot the two cuts of tofu with cheddar on one aspect. Include the vegetables and tomatoes.

Presently include several pickle cuts and near the sandwich collectively. Cut nook to corner

Dinner Recipes

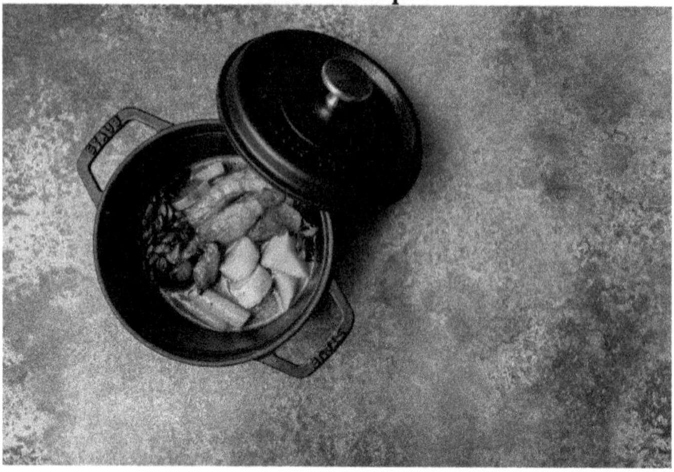

35 Pistachio Watermelon Steak

Preparation Time: 5 min.Cooking Time: 10 min.

Servings: 4Ingredients:
Microgreens

Pistachios choppedMalden sea salt

1 tbsp. olive oil, extra virgin1 watermelon
Salt to tasteDirections:
Begin by cutting the ends of the watermelon.

Carefully peel the skin from the watermelon along the white outer edge.

Slice the watermelon into 4 slices, approximately 2 inches thick.

Trim the slices, so they are rectangular in shape approximately 2 x4 inches.

Heat a skillet to medium heat add 1 tablespoon of olive oil.

Add watermelonsteaksandookuntiltheedgesbeginocaramelize.

Plate and top with pistachios and microgreens.Sprinkle with Malden salt.
Serve warm and enjoy!

Nutrition: Calories: 67 | Carbohydrates: 3.8 g | Proteins: 1.6 g Fats: 5.9 g

36 Collard greens 'n tofu

Preparation 15 minutesCooking: 20 minutes Servings: 4
Ingredients:

1 pounds of collard greens, rinsed, chopped1 cup water

1/2 pound of tofu, choppedSalt to taste
Pepper powder to taste

Crushed red chili to tasteDirection:
Place a large skillet over medium-high heat. Add oil. When the oil is heated, add tofu and cook until brown. Add rest of the ingredients and mix well.Cook until greens wilts and almost dry.

Lunch Recipes

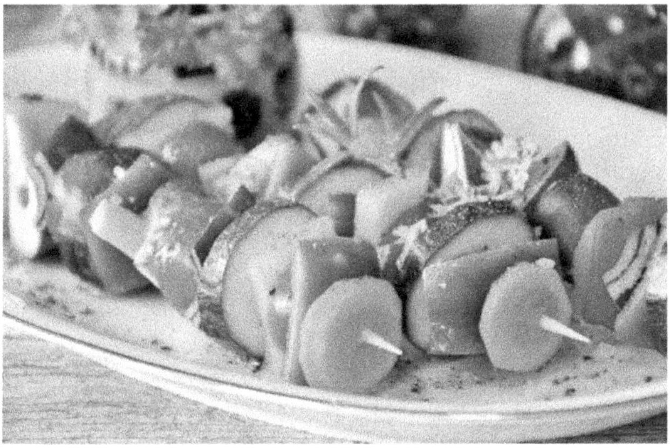

37 Thai Tofu And Quinoa Bowls

Preparation Time: 15 minutesCooking Time: 20 minutes Serving: 4
Ingredients:

3/4 cup (177 grams) quinoa, cooked

1 cup (236 grams) frozen edamame, thawed

12 ounces (175 grams) tofu, extra-firm, pressed

2 medium carrots, grated1 green onion, sliced
1/2 teaspoon minced garlic

2 teaspoons grated ginger 1/2 cup chopped cilantro 1/2 teaspoon red chili flakes1 tablespoon soy sauce
2 teaspoons agave syrup2 tablespoons lime juice
2 tablespoons peanut butter1 tablespoon water
4 teaspoons sesame seeds, toastedDirections:
Switch on the oven, set it to 400° F and let it preheat.Prepare the tofu: cut tofu into ¾-inch cubes.
Take a large baking sheet, line it with foil, spread tofu pieces on it,and bake for 20 minutes until golden brown, stirring halfway.

Prepare the drizzle: take a small bowl, place garlic, ginger, chili flakes, soy sauce, agave syrup, butter, lime, and water in it and then whisk until combined.

After tofu gets cooked, let it cool for 10 minutes and transfer into a large bowl.

Add carrot, green onions, cilantro, cabbage, and edamame, drizzle with

the prepared dressing and sprinkle with sesame seeds.
Mix quinoa with salad and serve.

Nutrition: 330 Cal; 13 g Fat; 3 g Saturated Fat; 36 g Carbs; 7 g Fiber; 19 g Protein; 10 g Sugar;

38 Green Beans with vegan Bacon

Preparation Time: 15 minutesCooking Time: 20 minutes Servings: 8
Ingredients:

1 slices of vegan bacon, chopped1 shallot, chopped
24 oz. green beans

Salt and pepper to taste

½ teaspoon smoked paprika1 teaspoon lemon juice
2 teaspoons vinegar

Direction

Preheat your oven to 450 degrees F.

Add the bacon in the baking pan and roast for 5 minutes.Stir in the shallot and beans.
Season with salt, pepper and paprika.Roast for 10 minutes.
Drizzle with the lemon juice and vinegar.Roast for another 2 minutes.
Nutrition:Calories:49Totalfat:1.2gSaturatedfat:0.4g Cholesterol: 3mgSodium: 92mgPotassium: 249mg Carbohydrates: 8.1gFiber: 3g Sugar: 4g Protein: 2.9g

39 Coconut Brussels Sprouts

Preparation: 15 minutesCooking: 10 minutes Servings: 4
Ingredients: 1 lb. Brussels sprouts, trimmed and sliced in half 2 tablespoons coconut oil ¼ cup coconut water tablespoon soy sauce Direction
In a pan over medium heat, add the coconut oil and cook theBrussels sprouts for 4 minutes.Pour in the coconut water.Cook for 3 minutes.Add the soy sauce and cook for another 1 minute.Nutrition: Calories: 114 Total fat: 7.1gSaturated fat: 5.7g Sodium: 269mgPotassium: 83mgarbohydrates: 1.1gFiber: 4.3g Sugar: 3g Protein: 4g

40 Cod Stew with Rice & Sweet Potatoes

Preparation: 30 minutesCooking: 1 hour Servings: 4 Ingredients:

1 cups water ¾ cup brown rice 1 tablespoon vegetable oil

1 tablespoon ginger, chopped1 tablespoon garlic, chopped
1 sweet potato, sliced into cubes1 bell pepper, sliced
1 tablespoon curry powderSalt to taste
15 oz. coconut milk4 cod fillets
2 teaspoons freshly squeezed lime juice3 tablespoons cilantro, chopped
Direction
Place the water and rice in a saucepan.

Bring to a boil and then simmer for 30 to 40 minutes. Set aside.Pour the oil in a pan over medium heat.

Cook the garlic for 30 seconds.

Add the sweet potatoes and bell pepper.Season with curry powder and salt. Mix well.

Pour in the coconut milk.Simmer for 15 minutes.
Nestle the fish into the sauce and cook for another 10 minutes.

Stir in the lime juice and cilantro.Serve with the rice.
Nutrition: Calories: 382 Total fat: 11.3g Saturated fat: 4.8g Cholesterol: 45mg Sodium: 413mg Potassium: 736mg Carbohydrates: 49.5g Fiber: 5.3g Sugar: 8g Protein: 19.2g

41 Avocado, Pine Nuts and Chard Salad

Preparation time: 5 minutesCooking time: 15 minutes Servings: 4
Ingredients:

1 pound swiss chard, roughly chopped2 tablespoons olive oil

1 avocado, peeled, pitted and roughly cubed2 spring onions, chopped
¼ Cup pine nuts, toasted

1 tablespoon balsamic vinegar Salt and black pepper to the taste
Directions:
Heat up a pan with the oil over medium heat, add the spring onions,pine nuts and the chard, stir and sauté for 5 minutes.

Add the vinegar and the other ingredients, toss, cook over mediumheat for 10 minutes more, divide into bowls and serve for lunch.

Nutrition: calories 120, fat 2, fiber 1, carbs 4, protein 8

42 Grapes, Avocado and Spinach Salad

Preparation time: 10 minutesCooking time: 0 minutes Servings: 4
Ingredients:

1 cup green grapes, halved2 cups baby spinach

1 avocado, pitted, peeled and cubedSalt and black pepper to the taste

2 tablespoons olive oil

1 tablespoon thyme, chopped

1 tablespoon rosemary, chopped1 tablespoon lime juice
1 garlic clove, minced

Directions:

In a salad bowl, combine the grapes with the spinach and the other ingredients, toss, and serve for lunch.

Nutrition: calories 190, fat 17.1, fiber 4.6, carbs 10.9, protein 1.7

43 Greens and Olives Pan

Preparation time: 10 minutesCooking time: 15 minutes Servings: 4
Ingredients:

4 spring onions, chopped2 tablespoons olive oil
½ cup green olives, pitted and halved

¼ cup pine nuts, toasted

1 tablespoon balsamic vinegar2 cups baby spinach
1 cup baby arugula

1 cup asparagus, trimmed, blanched and halvedSalt and black pepper to the taste

Directions:

Heat up a pan with the oil over medium high heat, add the spring onions and the asparagus and sauté for 5 minutes.

Add the olives, spinach and the other ingredients, toss, cook over medium heat for 10 minutes, divide between plates and serve for lunch.

Nutrition: calories 136, fat 13.1, fiber 1.9, carbs 4.4, protein 2.8

44 Cauliflower and Artichokes Soup

Preparation time: 10 minutesCooking time: 25 minutes Servings: 4
Ingredients:

1 pound cauliflower florets

1 cup canned artichoke hearts, drained and chopped2 scallions, chopped
2 tablespoons olive oil

2 garlic cloves, minced

6 cups vegetable stock

Salt and black pepper to the taste2/3 cup coconut cream
2 tablespoons cilantro, choppedDirections:
Heat up a pot with the oil over medium heat, add the scallions and the garlic and sauté for 5 minutes.

Add the cauliflower and the other ingredients, toss, bring to a simmerand cook over medium heat for 20 minutes more.

Blend the soup using an immersion blender, divide it into bowls and serve.

Nutrition: calories 207, fat 17.2, fiber 6.2, carbs 14.1, protein 4.7

Recipes For Main Courses And Single Dishes

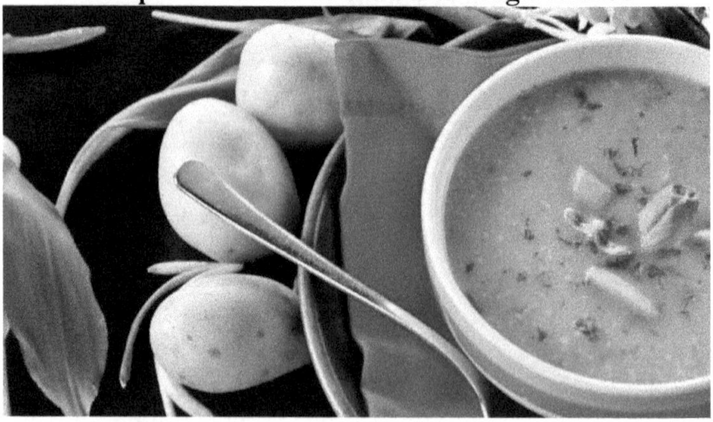

45 Mango Sticky Rice

Preparation Time: 35 MinutesCooking Time: 30 Minutes Servings: 3
Calories: 571

Protein: 6 Grams

Fat: 29.6 Grams

Carbs: 77.6 GramsIngredients:
½ Cup Sugar

1 Mango, Sliced

14 Ounces Coconut Milk, Canned

½ Cup Basmati RiceDirections:
Cook your rice per package instructions, and add half of your sugar. When cooking your rice, substitute half of your water for half of your coconut milk.

Boil your remaining coconut milk in a saucepan with your remaining sugar.

Boil on high heat until it's thick, and then add in your mango slices.

Interesting Facts: Mangos contain 50% of the daily Vitamin C you should consume which aid in bone and immune health.

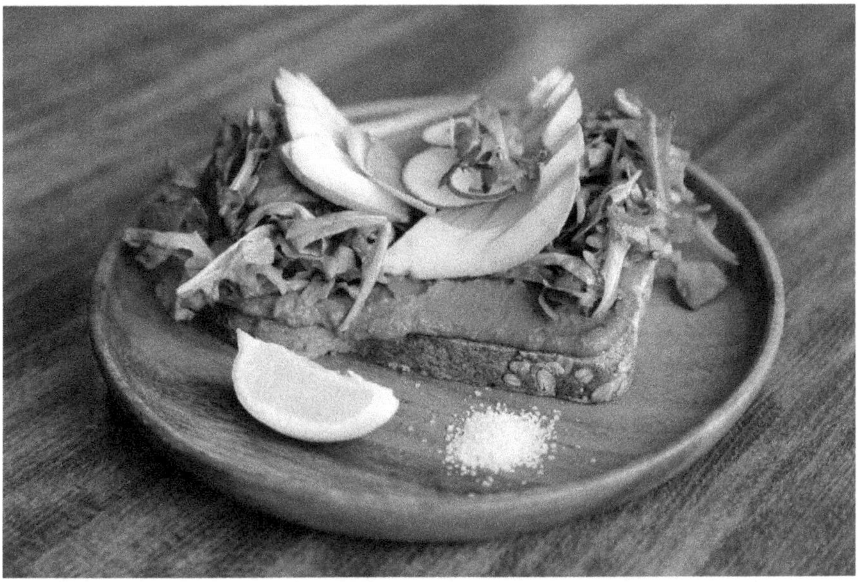

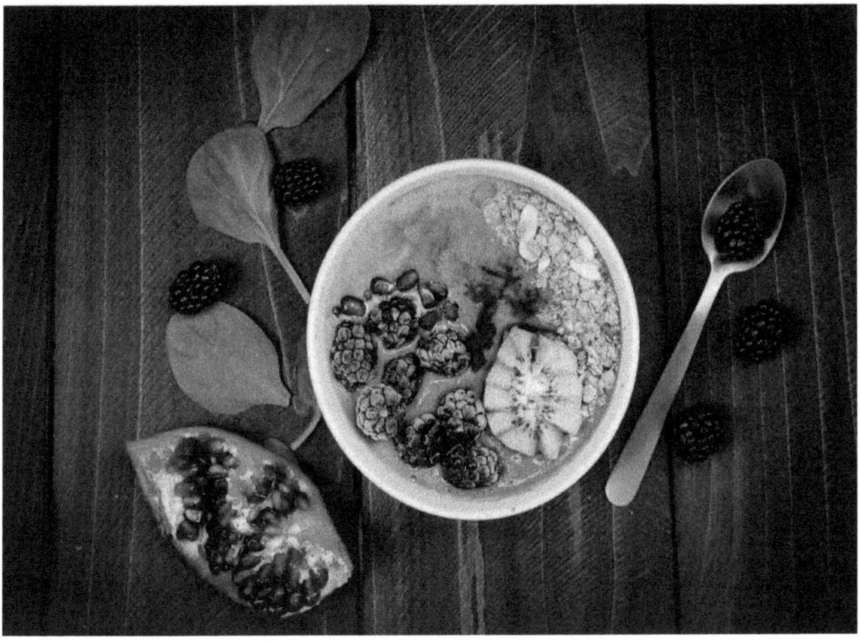

Nutrient-Packed Protein Salads

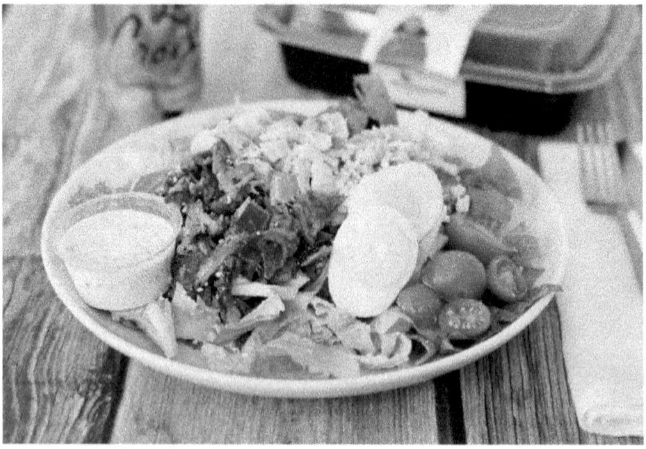

46 The Amazing Chickpea Spinach Salad

Preparation time: 10 minsCooking time: 10 mins
Ingredient: 1 can chickpeas (drained and rinsed)1 handful spinach
3.5 oz feta cheese (or similar cheese)1 small handful raisins
½ tbsp lemon juice (white or malt vinegar is also good)3 tsp honey 4 tbsp olive oil 0.5 - 1 tsp cumin1 pinch salt ½ tsp chili flakes (or dried cayenne pepper will do the trick nicely).

Directions:

Chop the cheese and add with the spinach and chickpeas to a large bowl Mix the honey, oil, lemon juice and raisins in a small bowl. Add the cumin, salt and pepper to the dressing bowl and mix well. Drizzle devilishly delicious dressing over the salad.

Flavour Boosters (Fish Glazes, Meat Rubs & Fish Rubs)

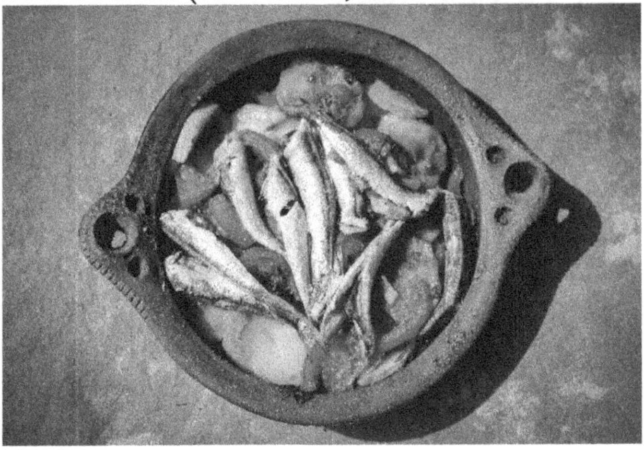

47 Southwestern Oregano Thyme Rub

This rub is a perfect blend of herbal, sweet, and earthy ingredients tomake your day truly special and delicious. If you wish to make your meat cuts less spicy, then you can adjust the quantity of chili powder.

Preparation Time: 5 min.Cooking Time: 5 min.
Servings: 11 tbs.

Ingredients:

Garlic powder - 2 tbs.Chili powder - 2 tbs. Dry mustard - 2 tbs.
Dried thyme- 1 tbs. Dried oregano - 1 tbs.Mild paprika - 1 tbs.
Ground coriander - 1 tbs.Ground cumin - 1 tbs.
Salt - 2 tsp.

Directions:

Mix all mentioned ingredients in your mixing bowl to make the oregano thyme rub. Gently mix all the ingredients using spatula or spoon to form an aromatic rub mixture.

Now, take your choice of meat cut and place it on a firm surface. Brush or rub the freshly made rub on it; pat gently for the rub to stick onto the surface. Turn the meat cut and repeat to spice up its other side. Repeat with other meat cuts.

The freshly rubbed meat is ready to be grilled or cooked!

48 Tangy Pepper & Thyme Rub

Transform your dry meats into full of citrusy, dark, and spicy flavors with this triple spice rub. The tangy thyme rub is quite easy to prepare and beautifully spices up your chicken, pork as well as beef.

Preparation Time: 5 min.Cooking Time: 0 min.
Servings: 2 tbs.

Ingredients:

Dried thyme - 1tbs.

Lime zest, finely grated – 1 tbs.

Sea salt and black pepper as requiredDirections:
Mix in all the ingredients in your mixing bowl to make the pepper and thyme rub. Gently mix all the ingredients using spatula or spoon to form an aromatic rub mixture.

Now, take your choice of meat cut and place it on a firm surface. Brush or rub the freshly made rub on it; pat gently for the rub to stick

onto the surface. Turn the meat cut and repeat to spice up its other side. Repeat with other meat cuts.

The freshly rubbed meat is ready to be grilled or cooked!

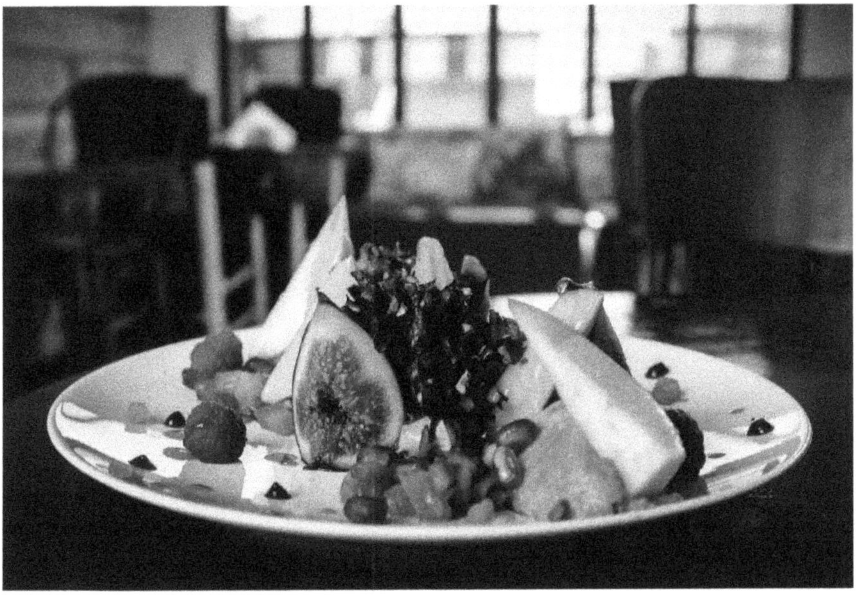

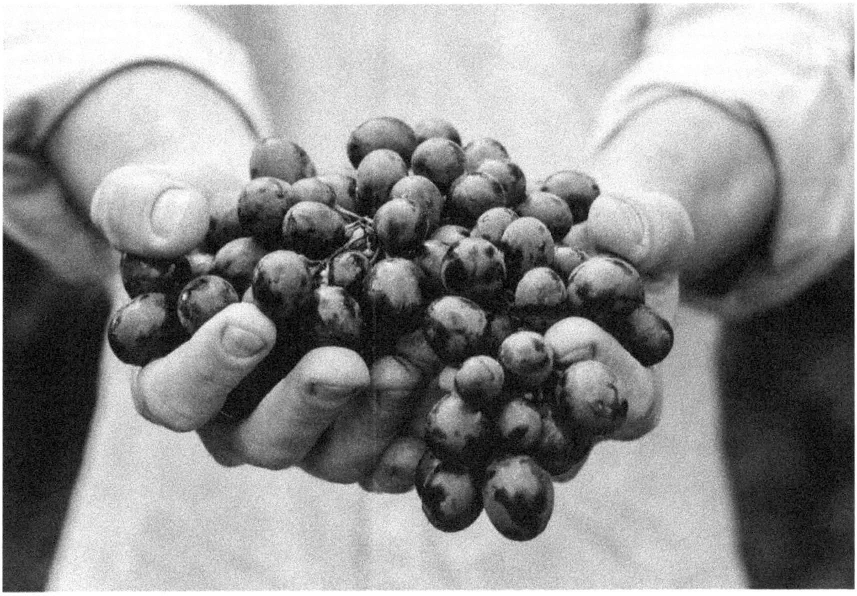

Sauce Recipes

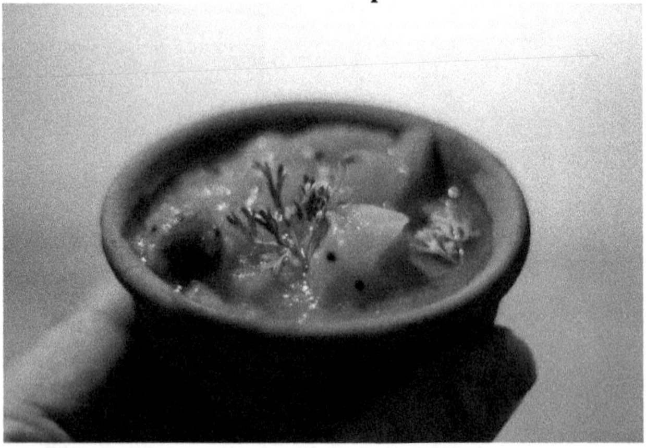

49 Coconut Sauce

Preparation time: 15 minutesCooking time: 15 minutes Servings: 3
Ingredients

½ cup red lentils, cooked 4 carrots, peeled, chopped
1 cup (250 ml) coconut milk, canned

3 tablespoons nutritional yeast

½ onion, diced

2 garlic cloves, minced Pepper and salt, to tasteDirections:
Boil the carrots for 10 minutes in a pan.

Blend the cooked carrots, lentils, onion, garlic, yeast and coconut milk in a blender until smooth. Stir in pepper and salt.

Pour the mixture into a saucepan and cook for 2 minutes, stirring frequently.

Pour the sauce over the cooked pasta or salad servers.

50 Vegan Bean Pesto

Preparation time: 5 minutesCooking time: 5 minutes Servings: 2
Ingredients

1 can (15 oz.) white beans, drained, rinsed 2 cups basil leaves, washed, dried
½ cup non-dairy milk 2 tablespoons olive oil
3 tablespoons nutritional yeast

1 garlic clove, peeled

Pepper and salt to tasteDirections:
Blend all the ingredients (except the seasonings) in a blender until smooth.

Sprinkle with pepper and salt to taste, then blend for 1 extra minute. Enjoy with pasta.

The Complete Plant Based Diet Cookbook 2021

2 Books in 1: 100+ Healthy and Delicious Vegan Recipes to Lose Weight Feel Great on a Budget

Frank Smith

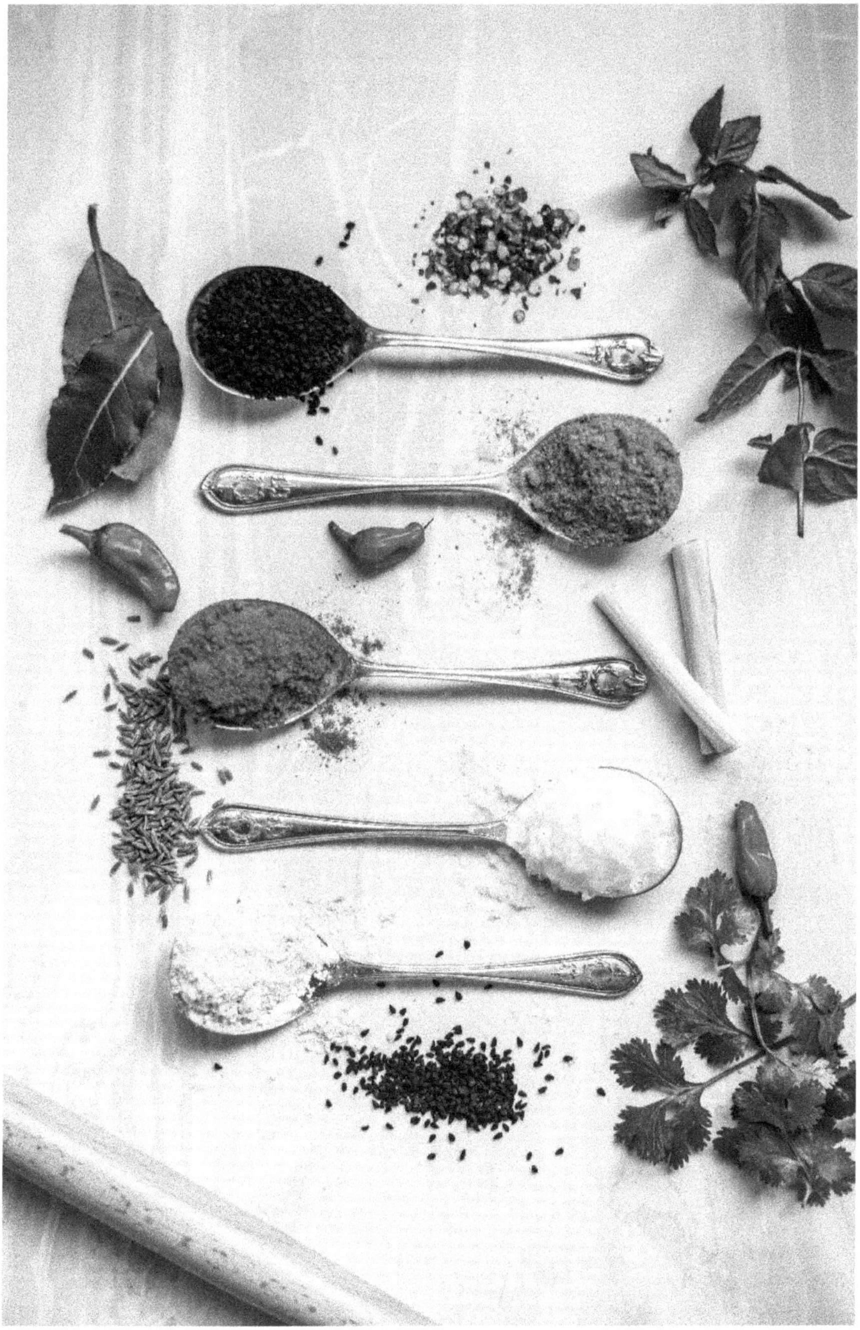

Breakfasts

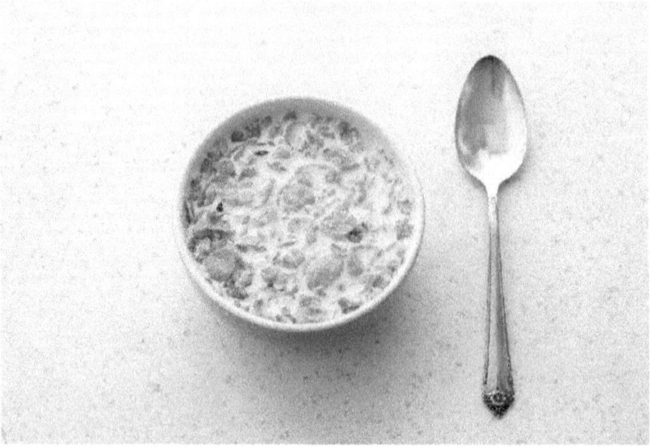

51 Oatmeal Fruit Shake

Preparation Time: 10 minutesCooking time: 0 minutes Servings: 2
Ingredients:

1 cup oatmeal, already prepared, cooled1 apple, cored, roughly chopped
1 banana, halved

1 cup baby spinach 2 cups coconut water2 cups ice, cubed
½ tsp ground cinnamon 1 tsp pure vanilla extractDirections:
Add all ingredients to a blender.

Blend from low to high for several minutes until smooth.

Nutrition: Calories 270 Carbohydrates 58 g Fats 1.5 g Protein 5 g

52 Amaranth Banana Breakfast Porridge

Preparation Time: 10 minutesCooking time: 25 minutes Servings: 8
Ingredients:

2 cup amaranth

2 cinnamon sticks

4 bananas, diced

2 Tbsp chopped pecans4 cups water
Directions:

Combine the amaranth, water, and cinnamon sticks, and banana in apot. Cover and let simmer around 25 minutes.

Remove from heat and discard the cinnamon. Places into bowls, and top with pecans.

Nutrition: Calories 330 Carbohydrates 62 g Fats 6 g Protein 10 g

53 Green Ginger Smoothie

Preparation time: 5 minutesCooking time: 5 minutes Servings: 2
Ingredients:

1 banana

½ apple sliced

1 orange sliced and peeled1 lemon juice
2 big spinach

1 tbsp. fresh ginger

½ cup almond milk

For the dressing: chia seeds, apple, raspberriesDirections:
Take a blender. Peel off and slice all fruits. Add banana, apple, orange, lime juice, ginger and spinach and blend them well until theyturn smooth. Now add almond milk and pulse again for a few seconds. Pour the smoothie into glasses and serve. You can add chia seeds, apple or raspberries for a smoothie bowl. Store it up to 8-10 hours in the refrigerator.

Nutrition: Calories 330 Carbohydrates 62 g Fats 6 g Protein 10 g

54 Chocolate Strawberry Almond Protein Smoothie

Preparation time: 10 mCooking time: 10 m Ingredients:
1 cup of organic strawberries

1 1/2 cup homemade almond milk 1 scoop chocolate protein powder 1 tablespoon organic coconut oil 1/4 cup organic raw almonds

2 tablespoon organic hemp seeds 1 tablespoon organic maca powderFor Garnish:
organic cacao nibs organic hemp seedsDirections:
Put all the ingredients inside a blender and beat until they are well combined.

Optional: Garnish with organic hemp seeds or organic cocoa beans.Enjoy it!
Nutrition: carbohydrates: 39 g calories: 720 Fat: 45 g sodium: 732g

protein: 44 g sugar: 12g

55 Apple and Cinnamon Oatmeal

Preparation time: 10 minutesCooking time:10 minutes Servings: 2
Ingredients

1¼ cups apple cider

1 apple, peeled, cored, and chopped

⅔ Cup rolled oats

1 teaspoon ground cinnamon

1 tablespoon pure maple syrup or agave (optional)Directions
In a medium saucepan, bring the apple cider to a boil over medium-high heat. Stir in the apple, oats, and cinnamon.

Bring the cereal to a boil and turn down heat to low. Simmer until the oatmeal thickens, 3 to 4 minutes. Spoon into two bowls and sweeten with maple syrup, if using. Serve hot.

56 13 bis. Mango Key Lime Pie Smoothie

Preparation time: 5 minutesCooking time: 0 minutes Servings: 1
Ingredients

¼ Avocado 1 cup baby spinach

½ Cup frozen mango chunks

1 cup unsweetened soy or almond milkJuice of 1 lime (preferably a key lime). 1 tablespoon maple syrup
Directions

Combine all the Ingredients in a blender and blend until smooth. Enjoy immediately.

57 Spiced Orange Breakfast Couscous

Preparation time: 10 minutesCooking time: 10 minutes Servings: 4
Ingredients

3 cups orange juice1½ cups couscous
1 teaspoon ground cinnamon

¼ Teaspoon ground cloves

½ Cup dried fruit, such as raisins or apricots

½ Cup chopped almonds or other nuts or seedsDirections
In a small saucepan, bring the orange juice to a boil. Add the couscous, cinnamon, and cloves and remove from heat. Cover the pan with a lid and allow to sit until the couscous softens, about 5 minutes.

Fluff the couscous with a fork and stir in the dried fruit and nuts. Serve immediately.

58 Fig & Cheese Oatmeal

Preparation Time: 10 minutesCooking Time: 0 minute Servings: 1
Ingredients:

½ cup water

½ cup rolled oatsPinch salt
2 tablespoons dried figs, sliced

2 tablespoons ricotta cheese

2 teaspoons agave syrup

1 tablespoon almonds, toasted and slicedDirections:
Put the water, oats and salt in a glass jar with lid.Shake to blend well. Refrigerate for up to 5 days.

Top with the remaining ingredients when ready to serve.

Nutrition: Calories: 294 Total fat: 8.5g Saturated fat: 2.3g Cholesterol: 10mg Sodium: 182mg Potassium: 362mg Carbohydrates: 47.5g Fiber: 6.6g Sugar: 16g Protein: 10.4g

59 Pumpkin Oats

Preparation: 10 minutesCooking: 0 minute Servings: 1
Ingredients:

½ cup rolle oats ½ cup almond milk ¼ cup ricotta cheese

2 tablespoons pumpkin puree1 tablespoon maple syrup
¼ teaspoon vanilla 1/8 teaspoon ground nutmegDirections:
Combine all the ingredients in a glass jar with lid.

Refrigerate for up to 5 days. Nutrition: Calories: 344 Total fat: 10g Saturated fat: 3.8g Cholesterol: 19mg Sodium: 179mg Potassium: 364mg Carbohydrates: 51.7g Fiber: 5.7g Sugar: 16g Protein: 13.3g

60 Apple Chia Pudding

Preparation time: 10 minutesCooking time: 5 minutes Servings: 04
Ingredients:

Chia Pudding:

4 tablespoons chia seeds1 cup almond milk
½ teaspoon cinnamonApple Pie Filling:

1 large apple, peeled, cored and chopped

¼ cup water

2 teaspoons maple syrupPinch cinnamon
2 tablespoons golden raisinsDirections:
In a sealable container, add cinnamon, chia seeds and almond milk, mix well.

Seal the container and refrigerate overnight.

In a medium pot, combine all apple pie filling ingredients and cook for 5 minutes.

Serve the chia pudding with apple filling on top.Enjoy.
Nutrition: Calories387TotalFat5.8gSaturatedFat4.2 g

Cholesterol 41 mg Sodium 154 mg Total Carbs 24.1 g Fiber 2.9 g

Sugar 3.1 g Protein 6.6 g

Soups, Salads, and Sides

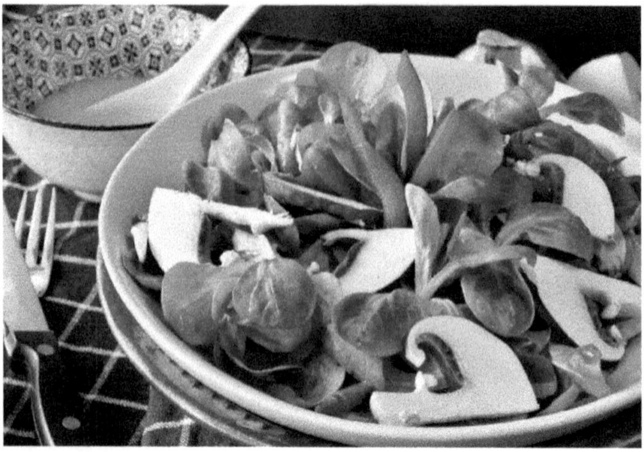

61 Garden PatchSandwichesonMultigrain Bread

Preparation time: 15 minutes Cooking time: 0 minutes Servings: 4 sandwiches Ingredients:

1pound extra-firm tofu, drained and patted dry1 medium red bell pepper, finely chopped

1 celery rib, finely chopped

3 green onions, minced

¼ cup shelled sunflower seeds

½ cup vegan mayonnaise, homemade or store-bought

½ teaspoon salt

½ teaspoon celery salt

¼ teaspoon freshly ground black pepper8 slices whole grain bread

4 (¼-inch) slices ripe tomato

4 lettuce leavesDirections:

Crumble the tofu and place it in a large bowl. Add the bell pepper, celery, green onions, and sunflower seeds. Stir in the mayonnaise, salt, celery salt, and pepper and mix until well combined.

Toast the bread, if desired. Spread the mixture evenly onto 4 slices of the bread. Top each with a tomato slice, lettuce leaf, and the remaining bread. Cut the sandwiches diagonally in half and serve.

62 Garden Salad Wraps

Preparation time: 15 minutesCooking time: 10 minutes Servings: 4 wraps Ingredients:
6 tablespoons olive oil

1-pound extra-firm tofu, drained, patted dry, and cut into ½-inch strips

1 tablespoon soy sauce

¼ cup apple cider vinegar

1 teaspoon yellow or spicy brown mustard

½ teaspoon salt

¼ teaspoon freshly ground black pepper3 cups shredded romaine lettuce
3 ripe roma tomatoes, finely chopped

1 large carrot, shredded

1 medium english cucumber, peeled and chopped

⅓ cup minced red onion

¼ cup sliced pitted green olives

4 (10-inch) whole-grain flour tortillas or lavash flatbreadDirections:
In a large skillet, heat 2 tablespoons of the oil over medium heat. Add the tofu and cook until golden brown, about 10 minutes. Sprinkle with soy sauce and set aside to cool.

In a small bowl, combine the vinegar, mustard, salt, and pepper with the remaining 4 tablespoons oil, stirring to blend well. Set aside.

In a large bowl, combine the lettuce, tomatoes, carrot, cucumber, onion, and olives. Pour on the dressing and toss to coat.

To assemble wraps, place 1 tortilla on a work surface and spread with about one-quarter of the salad. Place a few strips of tofu on the tortilla and roll up tightly. Slice in half

63 Marinated Mushroom Wraps

Preparation time: 15 minutes Cooking time: 0 minutes Servings: 2 wraps
Ingredients:
3 tablespoons soy sauce

3 tablespoons fresh lemon juice

11⁄2 tablespoons toasted sesame oil

2 portobello mushroom caps, cut into 1⁄4-inch strips 1 ripe hass avocado, pitted and peeled
2 cups fresh baby spinach leaves

1 medium red bell pepper, cut into 1⁄4-inch strips1 ripe tomato, chopped
Salt and freshly ground black pepper

Directions:

In a medium bowl, combine the soy sauce, 2 tablespoons of the lemon juice, and the oil. Add the portobello strips, toss to combine, and marinate for 1 hour or overnight. Drain the mushrooms and set aside.

Mash the avocado with the remaining 1 tablespoon of lemon juice.

To assemble wraps, place 1 tortilla on a work surface and spread with some of the mashed avocado. Top with a layer of baby spinach leaves. In the lower third of each tortilla, arrange strips of the soaked mushrooms and some of the bell pepper strips. Sprinkle with the

tomato and salt and black pepper to taste. Roll up tightly and cut inhalf diagonally. Repeat with the remaining ingredients and serve.

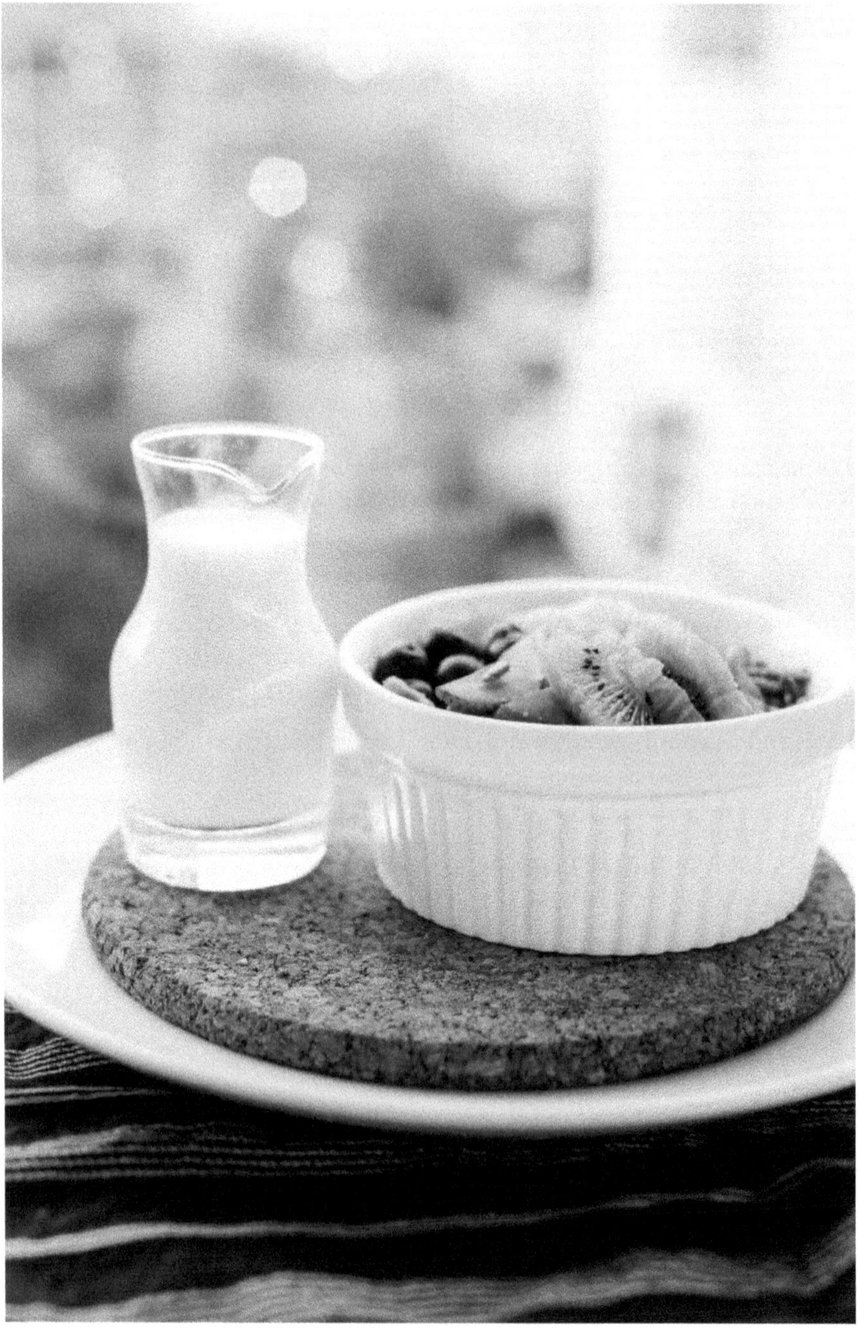

Entrées

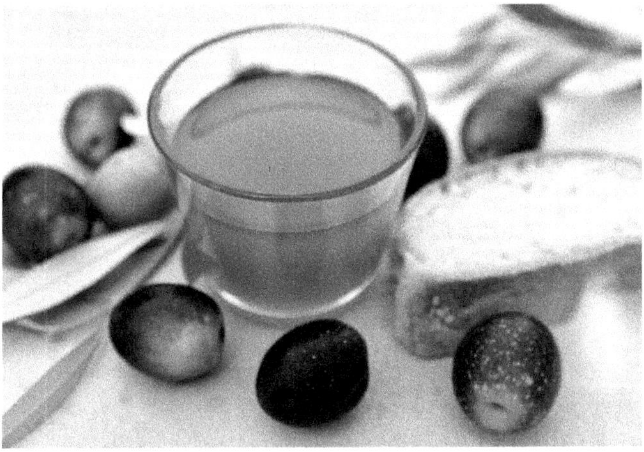

64 Homemade Trail Mix

Preparation time: 20 minutesCooking time: 20 minutes Servings: 2
Ingredients:

½ cup uncooked old-fashioned oatmeal

½ cup chopped dates

2 cups whole grain cereal

¼ cup raisins

¼ cup almonds

¼ cup walnutsDirections:
Mix all the ingredients in a large bowl.

Place in an airtight container until ready to use.

65 Nut Butter Maple Dip

Preparation time: 1 hourCooking time: 1 hour Servings:
Ingredients:

½ tablespoon ground flaxseed1 teaspoon ground cinnamon
½ tablespoon maple syrup

2 tablespoons cashew milk

¾ cups crunchy, unsweetened peanut butterDirections:
In a bowl, combine the flaxseed, cinnamon, maple syrup, cashew milk and peanut butter.

Use a fork to mix everything in. I stir it like I'm scrambling eggs. The mixture should be creamy. If it's too runny, add a little more peanut butter; if it's too thick, add a little more cashew milk.

Refrigerate for about an hour, covered and serve.

Smoothies and Beverages

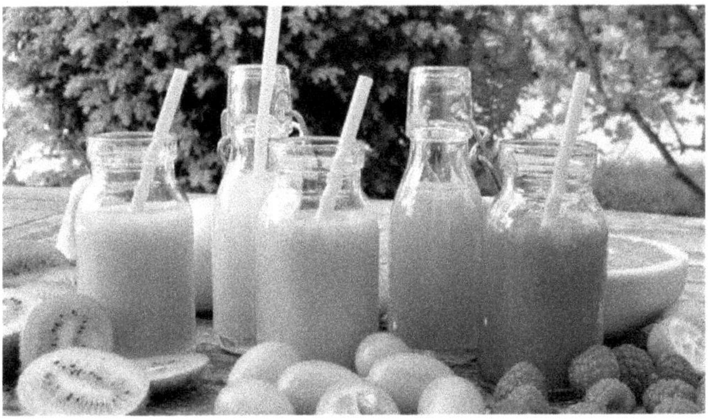

66 Kale & Avocado Smoothie

Preparation Time: 10 MinutesCooking time: 0 minute Servings: 1
Ingredients:

1 ripe banana

1 cup kale

1 cup almond milk

¼ avocado

1 tbsp. chia seeds2 tsp. honey
1 cup ice cubes

Direction:

Blend all the ingredients until smooth.

Nutrition: Calories 343 Total Fat 14 gSaturated Fat 2 g Cholesterol 0 mgSodium 199 mgTotal Carbohydrate 55 g Dietary Fiber 12 g Protein 6 gTotal Sugars 29 gPotassium 1051mg

67 Coconut & Strawberry Smoothie

Preparation Time: 10 MinutesCooking Time: 0 minutes Serves: 1
Calories: 278

Protein: 14 Grams

Fat: 2 Grams

Carbs: 57 GramsIngredients:
1 Cup Strawberries, Frozen & Thawed Slightly

1 Ripe Banana, Sliced & Frozen

½ Cup Coconut Milk, Light

½ Cup Vegan Yogurt

1 Tablespoon Chia Seeds

1 Teaspoon Lime juice, Fresh4 Ice Cubes
Directions:

Blend everything together until smooth, and serve immediately.

68 Pumpkin Chia Smoothie

Preparation Time: 5 MinutesCooking Time: 0 minutes Serves: 1
Calories: 726

Protein: 5.5 Grams

Fat: 69.8 Grams

Carbs: 15 GramsIngredients:
3 Tablespoons Pumpkin Puree

1 Tablespoon MCT Oil

¾ Cup Coconut Milk, Full Fat

½ Avocado, Fresh

1 Teaspoon Vanilla, Pure

½ Teaspoon Pumpkin Pie SpiceDirections:
Combine all ingredients together until blended.

69 Mini Berry Tarts

Preparation Time: 35 minutes + 1 hour chillingServings: 4
Tickle-sized berries-filled with surprises, oh so delicious! Also so delicious that you can't stop having them.

Ingredients

For the piecrust:

4 tbsp flax seed powder + 12 tbsp water

1/3 cup whole-wheat flour + more for dusting

½ tsp salt

¼ cup plant butter, cold and crumbled3 tbsp pure malt syrup
1 ½ tsp vanilla extractFor the filling:
6 oz cashew cream

6 tbsp pure date sugar

¾ tsp vanilla extract

1 cup mixed frozen berriesDirections
Preheat the oven to 350 F and grease a mini pie pans with cooking spray.

In a medium bowl, mix the flax seed powder with water and allow soaking for 5 minutes.

In a large bowl, combine the flour and salt. Add the butter and usingan electric hand mixer, whisk until crumbly. Pour in the flax egg, malt syrup, vanilla, and mix until smooth dough forms.

Flatten the dough on a flat surface, cover with plastic wrap, and refrigerate for 1 hour.

After, lightly dust a working surface with some flour, remove the dough onto the surface, and using a rolling pin, flatten the dough into a 1-inch diameter circle,

Use a large cookie cutter, cut out rounds of the dough and fit into thepie pans. Use a knife to trim the edges of the pan. Lay a parchment paper on the dough cups, pour on some baking beans and bake in the oven until golden brown, 15 to 20 minutes.

Remove the pans from the oven, pour out the baking beans, and allow cooling.

In a medium bowl, mix the cashew cream, date sugar, and vanilla extract.

Divide the mixture into the tart cups and top with berries. Serve immediately.

Nutritional info per serving

Calories 545 | Fats 33.5g| Carbs 53.6g | Protein 10.6g

70 Mixed Nut Chocolate Fudge

Preparation Time: 2 hours 10 minutes

Servings: 4

A recipe for chocolate fudge that takes just 10 minutes to make and requires ingredients that are readily available.

Ingredients

3 cups unsweetened chocolate chips

¼ cup thick coconut milk

1 ½ tsp vanilla extractA pinch salt
1 cup chopped mixed nuts

Directions

Line a 9-inch square pan with baking paper and set aside.

Melt the chocolate chips, coconut milk, and vanilla in a medium pot over low heat.

Mix in the salt and nuts until well distributed and pour the mixture into the square pan.

Refrigerate for at least for at least 2 hours.

Remove from the fridge, cut into squares and serve. Nutritional info per serving
Calories 907 | Fats 31.5g| Carbs 152.1g | Protein 7.7g

71 Date Cake Slices

Preparation Time: 1 hour 20 minutes

Servings: 4

With a slightly thick yet fluffy texture, they're super soft.Ingredients
½ cup cold plant butter, cut in pieces, plus extra for greasing1 tbsp flax seed powder + 3 tbsp water
½ cup whole-wheat flour, plus extra for dusting

¼ cup chopped pecans and walnuts1 tsp baking powder
1 tsp baking soda

1 tsp cinnamon powder

1 tsp salt

1/3 cup water

1/3 cup pitted dates, chopped

½ cup pure date sugar1 tsp vanilla extract
¼ cup pure date syrup for drizzling.

Directions

Preheat the oven to 350 F and lightly grease a round baking dish with some plant butter.

In a small bowl, mix the flax seed powder with water and allow thickening for 5 minutes to make the flax egg.

In a food processor, add the flour, nuts, baking powder, baking soda, cinnamon powder, and salt. Blend until well combined.

Add the water, dates, date sugar, and vanilla. Process until smooth with tiny pieces of dates evident.

Pour the batter into the baking dish and bake in the oven for 1 hour and 10 minutes or until a toothpick inserted comes out clean. Remove the dish from the oven, invert the cake onto a servingplatter to cool, drizzle with the date syrup, slice, and serve.

Nutritional info per serving

Calories 850 | Fats 61.2g| Carbs 65.7g | Protein 12.8g

72 Chocolate Mousse Cake

Preparation Time: 40 minutes + 6 hours 30 minutes chillingServings: 4

Have a cake with a basic mousse of chocolate and tell me how youfeel.

Ingredients

2/3 cup toasted almond flour

¼ cup unsalted plant butter, melted

2 cups unsweetened chocolate bars, broken into pieces2 ½ cups coconut cream

Fresh raspberries or strawberries for toppingDirections

Lightly grease a 9-inch springform pan with some plant butter andset aside.

Mix the almond flour and plant butter in a medium bowl and pour the mixture into the springform pan. Use the spoon to spread and press the mixture into the bottom of the pan. Place in the refrigerator tofirm for 30 minutes.

Meanwhile, pour the chocolate in a safe microwave bowl and meltfor 1 minute stirring every 30 seconds.

Remove from the microwave and mix in the coconut cream and maple syrup.

Remove the cake pan from the oven, pour the chocolate mixture on top making to sure to shake the pan and even the layer. Chill further for 4 to 6 hours.

Take out the pan from the fridge, release the cake and garnish with the raspberries or strawberries.

Slice and serve. Nutritional info per serving

Calories 608 | Fats 60.5g| Carbs 19.8g | Protein 6.3g

Snacks and Desserts

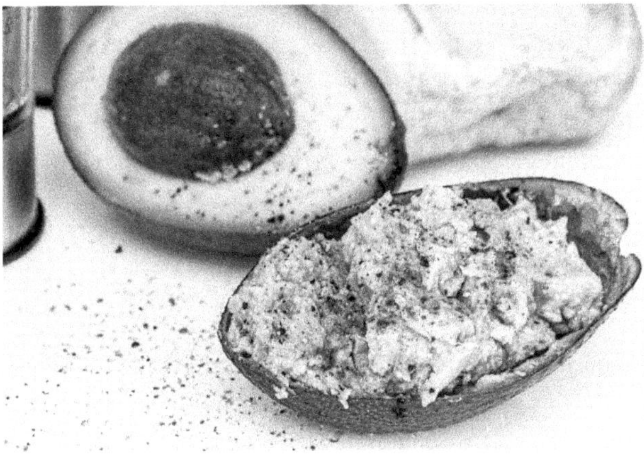

73 Nori Snack Rolls

Preparation Time: 5 minutesCooking time: 10 minutes Servings: 4 rolls
Ingredients

2 tablespoons almond, cashew, peanut, or others nut butter2 tablespoons tamari, or soy sauce
4 standard nori sheets

1 mushroom, sliced

1 tablespoon pickled ginger

½ cup grated carrotsDirections
Preparing the Ingredients. Preheat the oven to 350°F.
Mix together the nut butter and tamari until smooth and very thick. Lay out a nori sheet, rough side up, the long way.

Spread a thin line of the tamari mixture on the far end of the nori sheet, from side to side. Lay the mushroom slices, ginger, andcarrots in a line at the other end (the end closest to you).

Fold the vegetables inside the nori, rolling toward the tahini mixture, which will seal the roll. Repeat to make 4 rolls.

Put on a baking sheet and bake for 8 to 10 minutes, or until the rolls are slightly browned and crispy at the ends. Let the rolls cool for a few minutes, then slice each roll into 3 smaller pieces.

Nutrition: Calories: 79; Total fat: 5g; Carbs: 6g; Fiber: 2g; Protein: 4g

74 Risotto Bites

Preparation Time: 15 minutesCooking time: 20 minutes Servings: 12 bites
Ingredients
½ cup panko bread crumbs1 teaspoon paprika
1 teaspoon chipotle powder or ground cayenne pepper

1½ cups cold Green Pea RisottoNonstick cooking spray Directions
Preparing the Ingredients. Preheat the oven to 425°F.
Line a baking sheet with parchment paper.

On a large plate, combine the panko, paprika, and chipotle powder. Set aside.

Roll 2 tablespoons of the risotto into a ball.

Gently roll in the bread crumbs, and place on the prepared baking sheet. Repeat to make a total of 12 balls.

Spritz the tops of the risotto bites with nonstick cooking spray and bake for 15 to 20 minutes, until they begin to brown. Cool completely before storing in a large airtight container in a single layer (add a piece of parchment paper for a second layer) or in a plastic freezer bag.

Nutrition: Calories: 100; Fat: 2g; Protein: 6g; Carbohydrates: 17g; Fiber: 5g; Sugar: 2g; Sodium: 165 mg

75 Jicama and Guacamole

Preparation Time: 15 minutesCooking time: 0 minutes Servings: 4
Ingredients

juice of 1 lime, or 1 tablespoon prepared lime juice

2 hass avocados, peeled, pits removed, and cut into cubes

½ teaspoon sea salt

½ red onion, minced 1 garlic clove, minced
¼ cup chopped cilantro (optional)

1 jicama bulb, peeled and cut into matchsticksDirections
Preparing the Ingredients.

In a medium bowl, squeeze the lime juice over the top of theavocado and sprinkle with salt.

Lightly mash the avocado with a fork. Stir in the onion, garlic, and cilantro, if using.

Serve with slices of jicama to dip in guacamole.

To store, place plastic wrap over the bowl of guacamole and refrigerate. The guacamole will keep for about 2 days.

76 Oven-baked Caramelize Plantains

Preparation time: 30 minutesCooking time: 17 minutes Servings: 4
Ingredients

4 medium plantains, peeled and sliced2 Tbsp fresh orange juice
4 Tbsp brown sugar or to taste

1 Tbsp grated orange zest

4 Tbsp coconut butter, meltedDirections
Preheat oven to 360 F/180 C.

Place plantain slices in a heatproof dish.

Pour the orange juice over plantains, and then sprinkle with brown sugar and grated orange zest.

Melt coconut butter and pour evenly over plantains. Cover with foil and bake for 15 to 17 minutes.
Serve warm or cold with honey or maple syrup.

77 Powerful Peas & Lentils Dip

Preparation time: 10 minutesCooking time: 0 minutes Servings: 4
Ingredients

4 cups frozen peas

2 cup green lentils cooked1 piece of grated ginger
1/2 cup fresh basil chopped1 cup ground almonds Juice of 1/2 lime
Pinch of salt

4 Tbsp sesame oil

1/4 cup Sesame seedsDirections
Place all ingredients in a food processor or in a blender.

Blend until all ingredients combined well.

Keep refrigerated in an airtight container up to 4 days.

78 Protein "Raffaello" Candies

Preparation time: 15 minutesCooking time: 0 minutes Servings: 12
Ingredients

1 1/2 cups desiccated coconut flakes1/2 cup coconut butter softened
4 Tbsp coconut milk canned

4 Tbs coconut palm sugar (or granulated sugar) 1 tsp pure vanilla extract1 Tbsp vegan protein powder (pea or soy)15 whole almonds
Directions

Put 1 cup of desiccated coconut flakes, and all remaining ingredientsin the blender (except almonds), and blend until soft.

If your dough is too thick, add some coconut milk. In a bowl, add remaining coconut flakes.
Coat every almond in one tablespoon of mixture and roll into a ball. Roll each ball in coconut flakes.
Chill in the fridge for several hours.

79 Roasted Cauliflower

Preparation Time: 30 MinutesCooking Time: 20 Minutes Servings: 4
Ingredients:

Olive Oil (1 T.) Cauliflower (1, Chopped)Salt (to Taste)

Smoked Paprika (2 t.)Parsley (2 T.) Directions:
If you like to snack, it is better to have healthier options at hand. You'll want to start this recipe off by prepping your oven to 450.

As this warms up, place the cauliflower florets into a large mixing bowl and toss with the olive oil, salt, and smoked paprika. Once this is complete, lay it across a baking sheet and pop it into the oven for 20 minutes.

When the cauliflower is cooked to your liking, remove from the oven, top with parsley, and you are all set.

Nutrition: Calories: 70 Proteins: 3g Carbs: 8g Fats: 5g

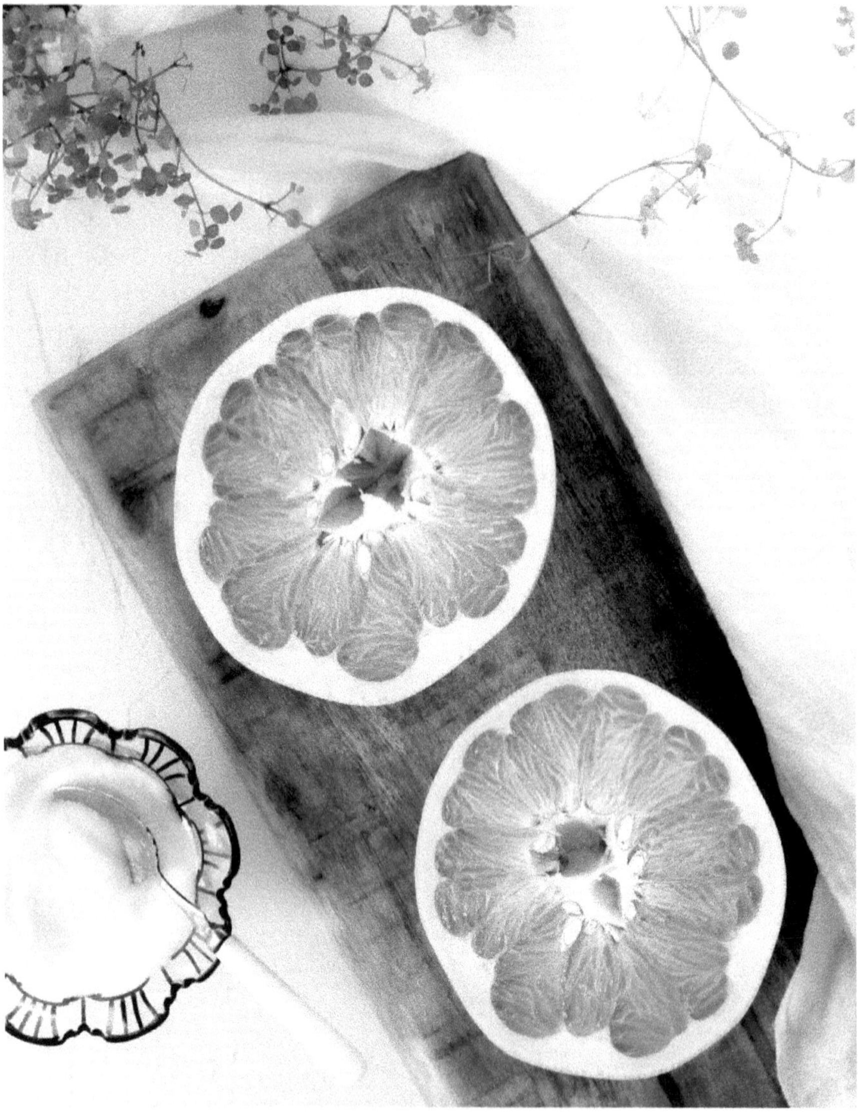

Dinner Recipes

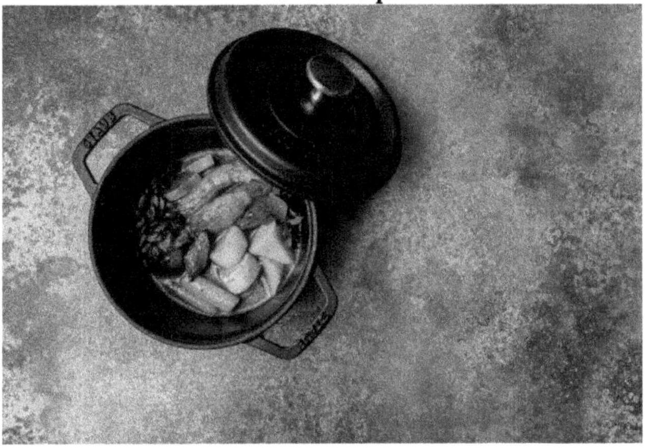

80 Cauliflower Steak Kicking Corn

Preparation: 30 min.Cooking: 60 min.Servings: 6

Ingredients:

2 t. capers, drained 4 scallions, chopped1 red chili, minced
¼ c. vegetable oil

2 ears of corn, shucked2 big cauliflower heads Salt and pepper to taste
Directions:
Heat the oven to 375 degrees.

Boil a pot of water, about 4 cups, using the maximum heat setting available.

Add corn in the saucepan, cooking approximately 3 minutes or until tender.

Drain and allow the corn to cool, then slice the kernels away from thecob.

Warm 2 tablespoons of vegetable oil in a skillet.

Combine the chili pepper with the oil, cooking for approximately 30 seconds.

Next, combine the scallions, sautéing with the chili pepper until soft. Mix in the corn and capers in the skillet and cook for approximately 1 minute to blend the flavors. Then remove from heat. Warm 1 tablespoon of vegetable oil in a skillet. Once warm, begin to place cauliflower steaks to the pan, 2 to 3 at a time. Season to your liking with salt and cook over medium heat for 3 minutes or until lightly browned. Once cooked, slide onto the cookie sheet and repeat step 5 with the remaining cauliflower.

Take the corn mixture and press into the spaces between the florets of the cauliflower.

Bake for 25 minutes. Serve warm and enjoy!
Nutrition: Calories: 153 | Carbohydrates: 15 g | Proteins: 4 g | Fats:10 g

81 Green beans stir fry

Preparation time 30 minutes

Cooking time: 10 minutesServings: 6-8 Ingredients:
1 1/2 pounds of green beans, stringed, chopped into 1 ½-inchpieces

1 large onion, thinly sliced4 star anise (optional)
3 tablespoons avocado oil

2 1/2 tablespoons tamari sauce or soy sauceSalt to taste
3/4 cup water

Direction:

Place a wok over medium heat. Add oil. When oil is heated, add onions and sauté until onions are translucent.

Add beans, water, tamari sauce, and star anise and stir. Cover andcook until the beans are tender.

Uncover, add salt and raise the heat to high. Cook until the water dries up in the wok. Stir a couple of times while cooking.

82 Mean bean minestrone

Preparation time: 45 minutesCooking time: 40 minutes Servings: 6
Protein content per serving: 9gIngredients
1 tablespoon (15 ml) olive oil

1/3 cup (80 g) chopped red onion

4 cloves garlic, grated or pressed

1 leek, white and light green parts, trimmed and chopped (about 4 ounces, or 113 g)

2 carrots, peeled and minced (about 4 ounces, or 113 g)2 ribs of celery, minced (about 2 ounces, or 57 g)
2 yellow squashes, trimmed and chopped (about 8 ounces, or 227 g) 1 green bell pepper, trimmed and chopped (about 8 ounces, or 227 g)
1 tablespoon (16 g) tomato paste1 teaspoon dried oregano
1 teaspoon dried basil

⅓ teaspoon smoked paprika

'¼ To ¼ teaspoon cayenne pepper, or to taste

2 cans (each 15 ounces, or 425 g) diced fire-roasted tomatoes4 cups (940 ml) vegetable broth, more if needed
3 cups (532 g) cannellini beans, or other white beans

2 cups (330 g) cooked farro, or other whole grain or pastaSalt, to taste
Nut and seed sprinkles, for garnish, optional and to tasteDirections:
In a large pot, add the oil, onion, garlic, leek, carrots, celery, yellow

squash, bell pepper, tomato paste, oregano, basil, paprika, and cayenne pepper. Cook on medium-high heat, stirring often until the vegetables start to get tender, about 6 minutes.

Add the tomatoes and broth. Bring to a boil, lower the heat, cover with a lid, and simmer 15 minutes.

Add the beans and simmer another 10 minutes. Add the farro and simmer 5 more minutes to heat the farro.

Note that this is a thick minestrone. If there are leftovers (which tasteeven better, by the way), the soup will thicken more once chilled.

Add extra broth if you prefer a thinner soup and adjust seasoning if needed. Add nut and seed sprinkles on each portion upon serving, if desired.

Store leftovers in an airtight container in the refrigerator for up to 5 days. The minestrone can also be frozen for up to 3 months.

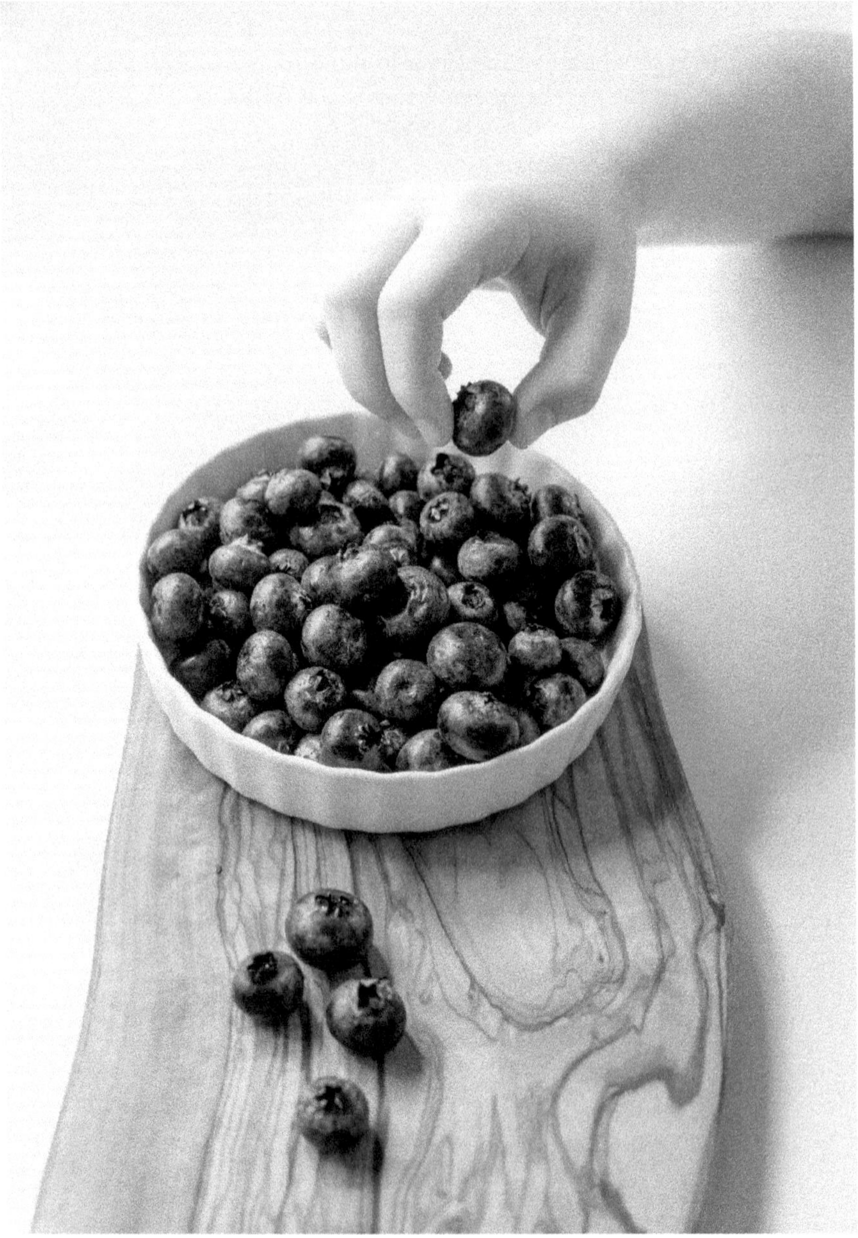

Lunch Recipes

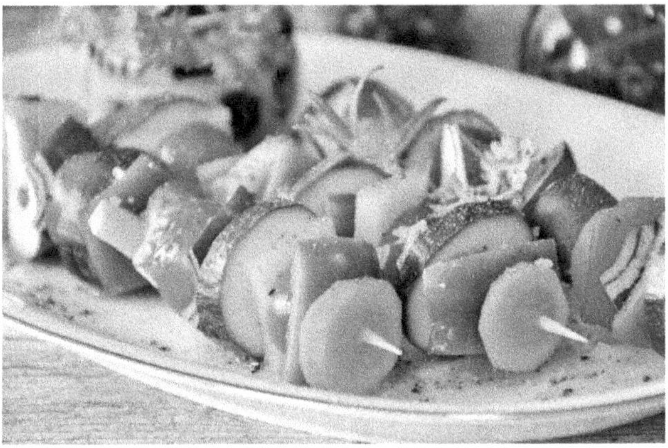

83 Chickpea And Edamame Salad

Preparation Time: 40 minutesCooking Time: 0 minutes Serving: 4
Ingredients:

For the Salad:

3 tablespoons dried cranberries 1/4 cup (59 grams) diced carrots
3/4 cup (177 grams) edamame soybeans 1/3 cup (78 grams) chopped green pepper30 ounces (850 grams) cooked chickpeas1/3 cup (78 grams) chopped red pepper 1/2 teaspoon minced garlic
For the Dressing:

1/4 teaspoon dried oregano1 teaspoon coconut sugar 1/4 teaspoon dried basil
1/3 teaspoon ground black pepper

1/3 teaspoon salt

1/4 teaspoon dried rosemary1 teaspoon white vinegar
2 tablespoons grape seed oil2 tablespoons olive oil Directions:
Preparethe salad: takealargesaladbowl, place allsalad ingredients in it and then toss until properly mixed.

Preparehe dressing:takeasmall bowl,placealldressingingredients in it and then whisk until combined.

Drizzle dressing over salad and toss until well mixed.

Place the salad bowl in the refrigerator for at least 30 minutes until chilled, then serve.

Nutrition: 119.6 Cal; 1.9 g Fat; 0.1 g Saturated Fat; 20.8 g Carbs; 4.8 g Fiber; 6 g Protein; 1.1 g Sugar;

84 Cauliflower Salad

Preparation Time: 20 minutesCooking Time: 15 minutes Servings: 4
Ingredients:

8 cups cauliflower florets

5 tablespoons olive oil, dividedSalt and pepper to taste
1 cup parsley

1 clove garlic, minced

2 tablespoons lemon juice

¼ cup almonds, toasted and sliced3 cups arugula
2 tablespoons olives, sliced

¼ cup feta, crumbledDirection
Preheat your oven to 425 degrees F.

Toss the cauliflower in a mixture of 1 tablespoon olive oil, salt and pepper.Place in a baking pan and roast for 15 minutes.Put the parsley, remaining oil, garlic, lemon juice, salt and pepper ina blender.Pulse until smooth.

Place the roasted cauliflower in a salad bowl.

Stir in the rest of the ingredients along with the parsley dressing.

Nutrition: Calories: 198 Total fat: 16.5g Saturated fat: 3g Cholesterol: 6mg Sodium: 3mg Potassium: 570mg Carbohydrates: 10.4g Fiber: 4.1g Sugar: 4g Protein: 5.4g

85 Garlic Mashed Potatoes & Turnips

Preparation: 20 minutesCooking: 30 minutes Servings: 8
Ingredients:

1 head garlic 1 teaspoon olive oil lb. turnips, sliced into cubes lb. potatoes, sliced into cubes

½ cup almond milk

½ cup vegan parmesan cheese, grated1 tablespoon fresh thyme, chopped

2 tablespoon fresh chives, chopped2 tablespoons vegan butter
Salt and pepper to tasteDirection
Preheat your oven to 375 degrees F.Slice the tip off the garlic head.
Drizzle with a little oil and roast in the oven for 45 minutes.

Boil the turnips and potatoes in a pot of water for 30 minutes or until tender.

Add all the ingredients to a food processor along with the garlic. Pulse until smooth.

Nutrition: Calories: 141 Total fat: 3.2g Saturated fat: 1.5g Cholesterol: 7mg Sodium: 284mg Potassium: 676mgCarbohydrates: 24.6g Fiber: 3.1g Sugar: 4g Protein: 4.6g

86 Pulled "Pork" Sandwiches

This pulled "pork" is the perfect dish to make ahead. Prepare the mushrooms and coat them in the sauce and then you can store them chilled in the cold-storage box or the icebox. If you prepare a large amount to keep in the icebox, you will always have some on hand for sandwiches, pizza, nachos, or any other vegan-version of popular dishes that might be complemented by pulled "pork".

Preparation time: 40 minutesCooking Time: 35 minutes Servings: 3
Ingredients:

King oyster mushrooms* – 4 Barbecue sauce – .25 cup Olive oil – 2 tablespoons Sea salt – .25 teaspoon Garlic, minced – 2 cloves
Cayenne pepper – .25 teaspoonBread – 6 slices
Directions:

Start by setting your electric cooker to Fahrenheit 400 degrees.

While your electric cooker warms up, clean the mushrooms with a damp paper towel and then use two forks to shred both the caps and stems of the mushrooms into pieces resembling pulled pork. Place

the shredded mushrooms on a kitchen parchment-lined aluminum baking sheet.

Drizzle the mushrooms with half of the olive oil and then toss them with the seasoning and garlic until evenly coated. Allow the oyster mushrooms to roast until slightly crispy and browned about twenty minutes.

In a skillet, add the remaining tablespoon of olive oil, allowing it to warm over midway-elevated. Put the cooked mushrooms in the pan along with the barbecue sauce.

Cook the mushrooms in the sauce while stirring until the sauce is fragrant and warm, about three to five minutes. Top three slices of bread with this concoction and top with the remaining three slices. Cut the sandwiches in half before serving. Note:

*If you can't find king oyster mushrooms, then you can use three heaping cups of regular oyster mushrooms.

Nutrition: Calories 259

87 Coconut zucchini cream

Preparation time: 10 minutesCooking time: 25 minutes Servings: 4
Ingredients:

1 pound zucchinis, roughly chopped2 tablespoons avocado oil
4 scallions, chopped

Salt and black pepper to the taste6 cups veggie stock
1 teaspoon basil, dried

1 teaspoon cumin, ground3 garlic cloves, minced
¾ cup coconut cream

1 tablespoon dill, choppedDirections:
Heat up a pot with the oil over medium high heat, add the scallions and the garlic and sauté for 5 minutes.

Add the rest of the ingredients, stir, bring to a simmer and cook over medium heat for 20 minutes more.

Blend the soup using an immersion blender, ladle into bowls and serve.

Nutrition: calories 160, fat 4, fiber 2, carbs 4, protein 8

88 Zucchini and Cauliflower Soup

Preparation time: 10 minutesCooking time: 25 minutes

Servings: 4Ingredients:
4 scallions, chopped

1 teaspoon ginger, grated2 tablespoons olive oil

1 pound zucchinis, sliced

2 cups cauliflower florets

Salt and black pepper to the taste6 cups veggie stock
1 garlic clove, minced

1 tablespoon lemon juice1 cup coconut cream Directions:
Heat up a pot with the oil over medium heat, add the scallions, ginger and the garlic and sauté for 5 minutes.

Add the rest of the ingredients, bring to a simmer and cook over medium heat for 20 minutes.

Blend everything using an immersion blender, ladle into soup bowlsand serve.

Nutrition: calories 154, fat 12, fiber 3, carbs 5, protein 4

89 Chard soup

Preparation time: 10 minutesCooking time: 25 minutes Servings: 4
Ingredients:

1 pound Swiss chard, chopped

½ cup shallots, chopped 1 tablespoon avocado oil 1 teaspoon cumin, ground

1 teaspoon rosemary, dried1 teaspoon basil, dried

2 garlic cloves, minced

Salt and black pepper to the taste6 cups vegetable stock
1 tablespoon tomato passata

1 tablespoon cilantro, choppedDirections:
Heat up a pan with the oil over medium heat, add the shallots and the garlic and sauté for 5 minutes.

Add the swiss chard and the other ingredients, toss, bring to asimmer and cook over medium heat for 20 minutes more.

Divide the soup into bowls and serve.

Nutrition: calories 232, fat 23, fiber 3, carbs 4, protein 3

90 Eggplant and Olives Stew

Preparation time: 10 minutesCooking time: 30 minutes Servings: 4
Ingredients:

2 scallions, chopped

2 tablespoons avocado oil

2 garlic cloves, chopped 1 bunch parsley, chopped
Salt and black pepper to the taste

1 teaspoon basil, dried 1 teaspoon cumin, dried
2 eggplants, roughly cubed

1 cup green olives, pitted and sliced3 tablespoons balsamic vinegar
½ Cup tomato passataDirections:
Heat up a pot with the oil over medium heat, add the scallions, garlic,basil and cumin and sauté for 5 minutes.

Add the eggplants and the other ingredients, toss, cook over mediumheat for 25 minutes more, divide into bowls and serve.

Nutrition: calories 93, fat 1.8, fiber 10.6, carbs 18.6, protein 3.4

Recipes For Main Courses And Single Dishes

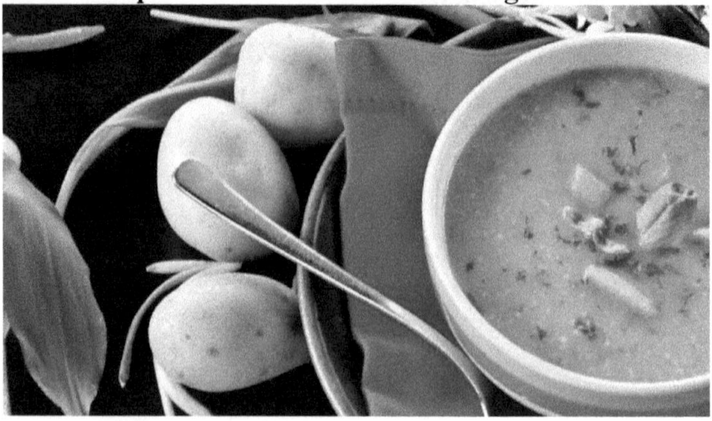

91 Pecan & Blueberry Crumble

Preparation Time: 40 MinutesCooking Time: 1 Hour Servings: 6
Calories: 381

Protein: 10 Grams

Fat: 32 Grams

Net Carbs: 20 GramsIngredients:
14 Ounces Blueberries

1 Tablespoon Lemon Juice, Fresh1 ½ Teaspoon Stevia Powder
3 Tablespoons Chia Seeds

2 Cups Almond Flour, Blanched

¼ Cup Pecans, Chopped 5 Tablespoon coconut Oil 2 Tablespoon Cinnamon Directions:
Mix together your blueberries, stevia, chia seeds and lemon juice,and place it in an iron skillet.

Mix ingredients while spreading it over your blueberries.

Heat your oven to 400, and then transfer it to an oven safe skillet, baking for a half hour.

Interesting Facts: Blueberries: These guys are a delectable treat thatis easily incorporated into many dishes. They are packed with antioxidants and Vitamin C. Bonus: Blueberries have been proven to promote eye health and slow macular degeneration.

92 Rice Pudding

Preparation Time: 1 Hour 35 Minutes Cooking Time: 1 Hour and 30 MinutesServings: 6
Ingredients:

1 Cup Brown Rice

1 Teaspoon Vanilla Extract, Pure

½ Teaspoon Sea Salt, Fine

½ Teaspoon Cinnamon

¼ Teaspoon Nutmeg3 Egg Substitutes
3 Cups Coconut Milk, Light

2 Cups Brown Rice, CookedDirections:
Blend all of your ingredients together before pouring them into a two quarter dish.

Bake at 300 for ninety minutes before serving.

Interesting Facts: Brown rice is incredibly high in antioxidants and good vitamins. It's relative, 14 white rice is far less beneficial asmuch of these healthy nutrients get destroyed during the process of milling. You can also opt for red and black rice or wild rice. The meal options for this healthy grain are limitless!

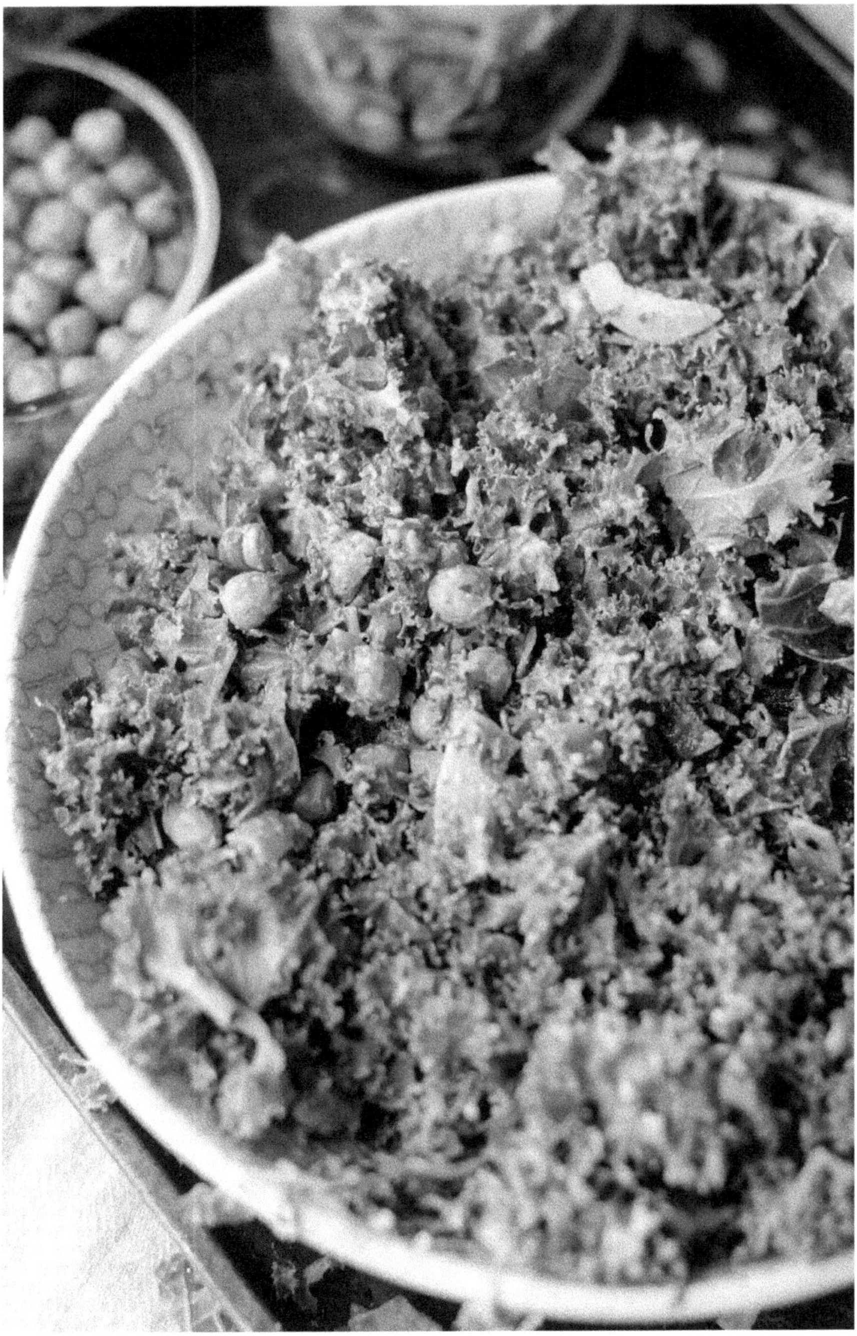

Nutrient-Packed Protein Salads

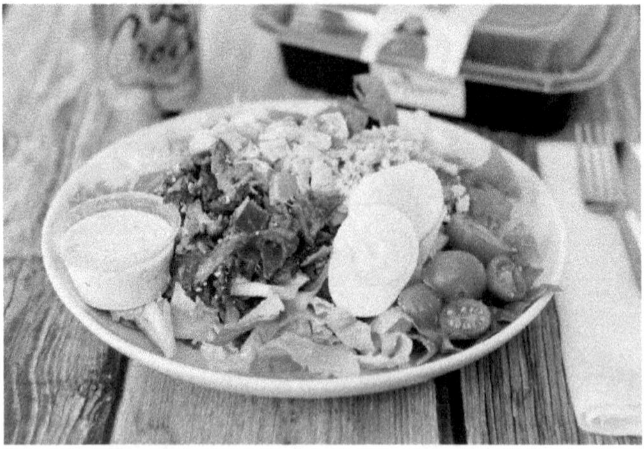

93 Chickpea, Red Kidney Bean And Feta Salad

Preparation time: 5 minsCooking time: 5 mins Ingredient:

1 can chickpeas

1 can red kidney beans

1 piece small of ginger grated or shredded1 medium onion diced
2- 3 cloves garlic

1 tbsp olive oil

A pinch of red chili flakes

3-4 spring onions green part only, chopped, scallions 1 cup chopped parsley OR coriander I used cilantro Juice of one lemon150 g feta cheese – almost half cup sizeSalt and Black pepper.

Directions:

Heat 1 tablespoon of olive oil and cook the onion till lightly golden. Do not overdo it and the onions should still be crunchy. Add garlic, ginger and chili and cook till the garlic is fragrant. Set aside to cool so it doesn't melt the feta when you mix it in. Drain the chickpeasand red kidney beans, rinse and place in the salad bowl. Add crumbled feta, spring onion, parsley (or coriander) and lemon juice, season with salt and pepper. Add the cooled onion and garlic mixtureand remaining oil and mix well.

94 Curried Carrot Slaw With Tempeh

Preparation: 10 minsCooking: 10 mins

Ingredient:

8 ounces tempeh, sliced into triangles 1/4 tsp liquid smoke (optional) 1 1/2 Tbsp maple syrup, grade B

1 tsp extra virgin olive oil or virgin coconut oil2-3 tsp tamari or 2 tsp soy sauce
1 Tbsp crushed raw walnuts4 cups shredded carrots
1 small onion, diced 1 Tbsp curry powder
1/4 tsp turmeric powder (for added turmeric power, optional) 1/8 tsp black pepper2 Tbsp tahini
1/4 cup fresh lemon juice sweet stuff: 1 – 1 1/2 Tbsp maple syrup + an optional handful orraisins

1/2 cup flat leaf parsley, finely chopped + some for garnish

a few pinches of cayenne for heat (optional) salt and pepper for carrot salad – to taste.

Directions:

Warm a skillet up over high heat and add in the coconut or olive oil. When oil is hot, add the tempeh triangles, tamari, maple and liquid smoke. Flip the tempeh around a bit to allow it to absorb the liquid. Cook for about 5 minutes, flipping the tempeh a few times throughout the cooking process. When tempeh is browned and edges blackened a bit, and all liquid absorbed, turn off heat. Sprinkle the walnut pieces and some black pepper over top the tempeh and set pan aside to keep triangles warm in skillet. In a large mixing bowl, add the carrots, tahini, lemon juice, spices, parsley, maple syrup, optional raisins and onion. Toss very well for a few minutes to marinate the carrots with the dressing. For a creamier salad, add another spoonful of tahini. To thin things out and make the salad zestier, add another splash of lemon juice or a teaspoon of apple cider vinegar. Finally, add salt and pepper to the carrot salad to taste. Pour the carrot salad in a large serving bowl and top with the tempeh. Serve right away or place in the fridge to serve in a few hours or up to a day later. The carrots will soften the longer they set in the fridge.

95 Black & White Bean Quinoa Salad

Preparation time: 15 minsCooking time: 15 mins Ingredient:

⅓ cup (75 mL) quinoa

1 can (19 oz/540 mL) black beans, drained and rinsed

1 can (19 oz/540 mL) navy beans, drained and rinsed1 cup (250 mL) diced cucumbers

¼ cup (50 mL) diced red onion

1 jalapeno pepper, seeded and minced (I've never used it and findthe dish spicy enough for me, but feel free to add it if you like things hot!)

¼ cup (50 mL) chopped fresh coriander (cilantro)

¼ cup (50 mL) vegetable oil (I use cold pressed extra-virgin olive oil)

2 tbsp (25 mL) lime juice

1 tbsp (15 mL) cider vinegar1 clove garlic, minced

½ tsp (2 mL) chili powder

1 tsp (5 mL) ground coriander

½ tsp (2 mL) dried oregano

¼ tsp (1 mL) salt

¼ tsp (1 mL) pepper.

Directions:

In saucepan of boiling salted ⅔ C water, cook quinoa until tender, about 12 minutes. Drain and rinse. Dressing: In large bowl, whisk together oil, lime juice, vinegar, garlic, chili powder, coriander, oregano, salt and pepper. Add quinoa, black beans, navy beans, cucumber, onion, jalapeño pepper and coriander; toss to combine.

96 Greek Salad With Seitan Gyros Strips

Preparation time: 5 mins

Cooking time: 5 minsIngredient: 4 tomatoes
1 punnet cherry tomatoes

1 1/2 crunchy cucumbers

1 big handful kalamata olives 1/2 Spanish onion finely sliced
1/4 stick of Cheesy mozzarella style cheese.Fresh oregano and mint
1/4 cup good quality extra virgin olive oil

2 Tablespoons vinegar (red wine or balsamic)1 teaspoon castor sugar
2 teaspoons mixed dried Italian herbs1 clove finely chopped garlic

1 teaspoon soy saucesalt
pepper.

Directions:

In a small frying pan, place gyros strips and fry until slightly blackened on the edges. Leave to cool. Cut up all your veggies roughly and place in a large bowl. Add olives, oregano, mint and chopped cheese. In a jar add all dressing ingredients. Shake welland taste. Combine the cooled gyros strips, salad and dressing and coat well.

97 Chickpea And Edamame Salad

Preparation time: 30 mins

Cooking time: 30 mins

Ingredient: 2 15.5oz each cans chickpea (garbanzo beans) rinsedand drained

3/4 cup edamame soy beans 1/3 cup chopped red pepper 1/3 cup chopped green pepper1/4 cup diced carrots
3 tablespoons dried cranberries1 garlic clove minced
Dressing

2 tablespoons grapeseed oil2 tablespoons olive oil
1 teaspoon white distilled vinegar1 teaspoon sugar
1/4 teaspoon dried oregano1/4 teaspoon dried basil
1/4 teaspoon dried rosemary

Salt and pepperDirections:
In a large bowl combine chickpeas, edamame, red pepper, green

pepper, carrots, dried cranberries, minced garlic and set aside. In a small bowl combine grapeseed oil, olive oil, vinegar, sugar, oregano, basil and rosemary. Whisk until blended. Pour dressing over chick peas and gently toss. Season with salt and pepper to taste. Chill for at least 30 minutes for flavors to blend. Serve chilled.

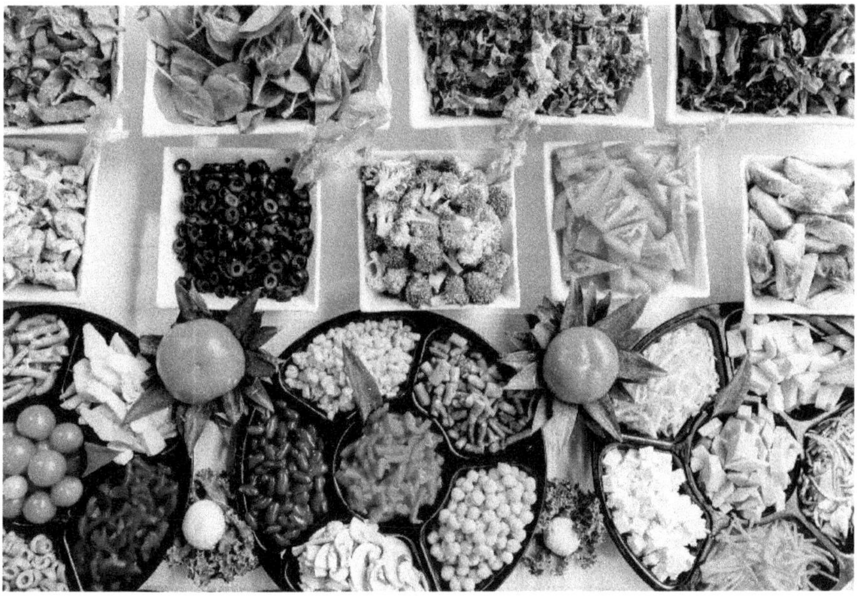

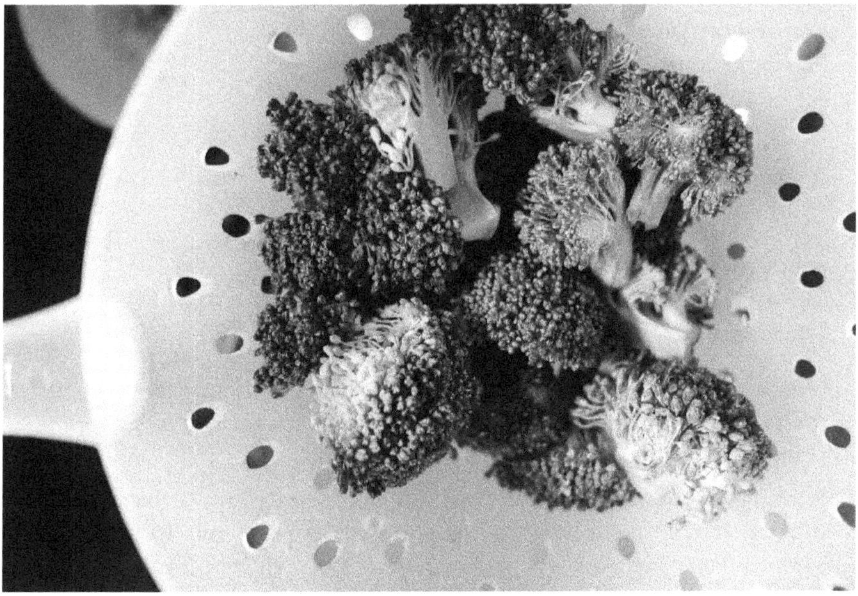

Flavour Boosters (Fish Glazes, Meat Rubs & Fish Rubs)

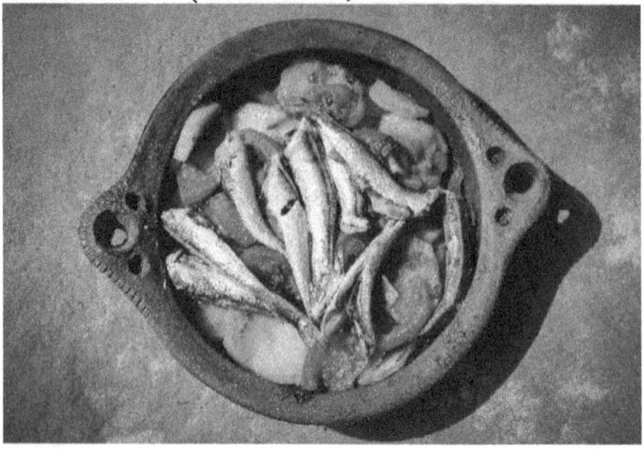

98 Mexican Cocoa Rub

Want to spice up your dry meats with savory Mexican flavors? Tryout my classy rub this weekend. Cocoa and espresso powder are a special addition to this Mexican style rub creating soothing spiced aroma.

Preparation Time: 5 min.Cooking Time: 5 min.
Servings: 9 tsp.

Ingredients:

Water – 1 tbs.

Cocoa, unsweetened – 1 tsp. Instant espresso powder – 2 tsp. Smoked paprika – 2 tsp.
Olive oil – 1 tsp. Ground cumin – 1 tsp.Salt – ¼ tsp.
Directions:

One by one, mix in all the ingredients in your mixing bowl to make the cocoa rub. Gently mix all the ingredients using spatula or spoon to form an aromatic rub mixture.

Now, take your choice of meat cut and place it on a firm surface. Brush or rub the freshly made rub on it; pat gently for the rub to stick to the surface. Turn the meat cut and repeat to spice up its other side. Repeat with other meat cuts.

Let your meat cuts adequately season for more rich flavors for a few hours in your refrigerator. Take them out, as they are ready to be cooked or grilled!

99 Juniper Sage Meat Rub

This unique meat rub has been crafted with quality by including numerous healthy herbs such as juniper berries, lay leaf, red pepper, etc. It delivers piney accent to the rub, which ultimately enhances the flavor of your favorite meat cuts.

Preparation Time: 5 min.Cooking Time: 5 min.
Servings: 8 tsp. Ingredients:

Bay leaf – 1 Black peppercorns - 1 tsp.Juniper berries - 2 tsp. Extra-virgin olive oil - 2 tbs. Crushed red pepper - ½ tsp.Kosher salt - ½ tsp.
Minced garlic – 1 cloveMinced sage leaves - 6Directions:
Mix in the bay leaf, red pepper, salt, peppercorns, and berries in yourspice blender, grinder or processor to make the juniper rub. Start processing or grinding the mixed spiced on "pulse" mode to ground.

Empty the mixed spice mixture in a bowl; mix in the sage leaves, oil, and garlic. Mix again well.

Now, take your choice of meat cut and place it on a firm surface. Brush or rub the freshly made rub on it; pat gently for the rub to stick to the surface. Turn the meat cut and repeat to spice up its other side. Repeat with other meat cuts.

The freshly rubbed meat is ready to be grilled or cooked!

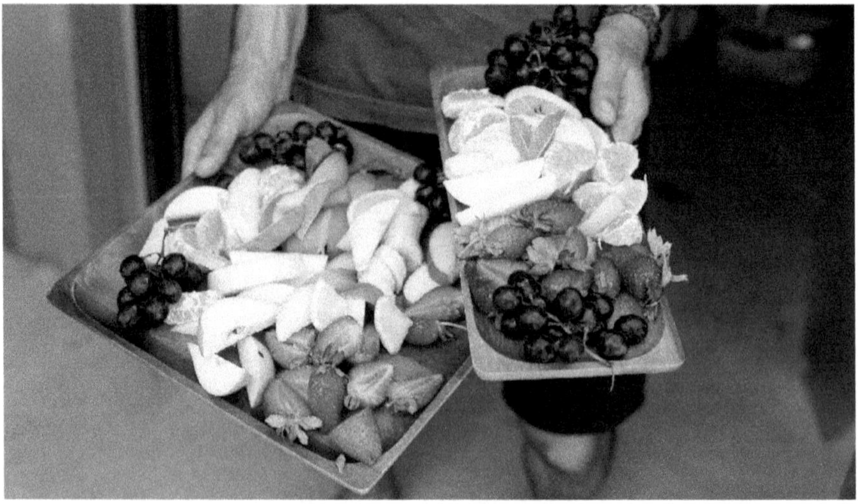

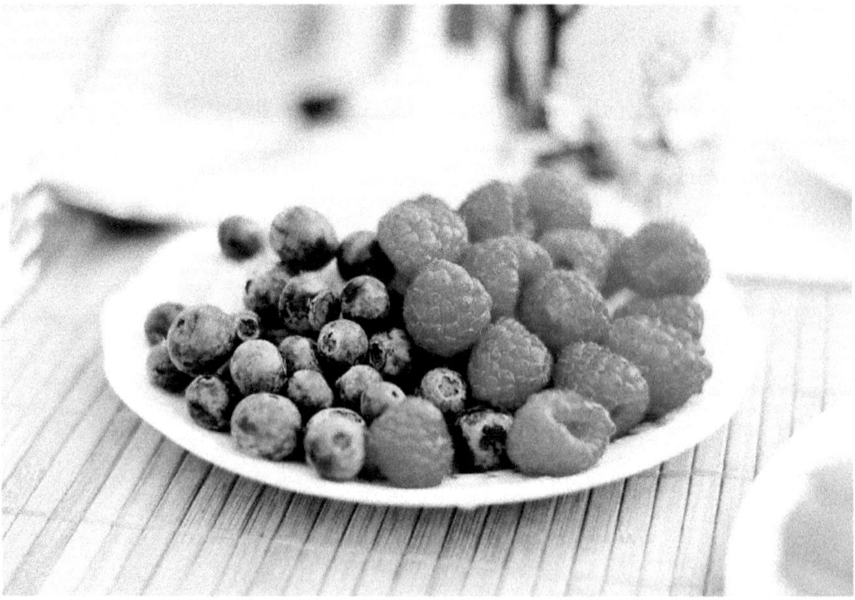

Sauce Recipes

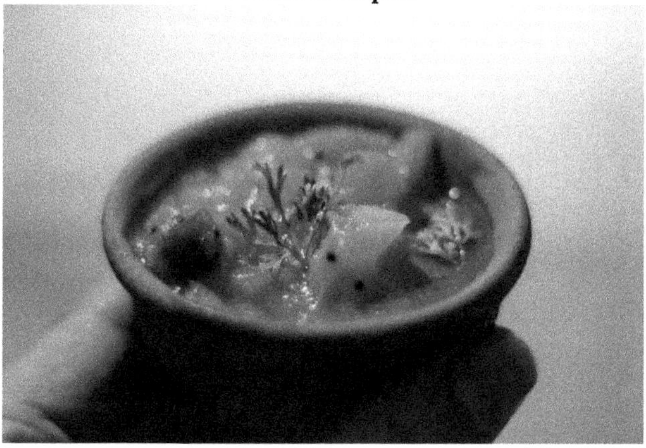

100 Coconut Sugar Peanut Sauce

Preparation time: 5 minutes Cooking time: 5 minute Servings: 1 ½ cups
Ingredients
4 tablespoons coconut sugar

6 tablespoons powdered peanut butter1 tablespoon chili sauce
2 tablespoons liquid aminos

¼ cup of water

1 teaspoon lime juice

½ teaspoon ginger powderDirections:
In a bowl, combine all the ingredients until properly combined. Serve as a topping for the salad or other dishes.Store in a fridge.

The Plant-based Cookbook

Healthy and Flavorful Recipes to Kick-Start your Health & Live Your Best

Frank Smith

Breakfasts

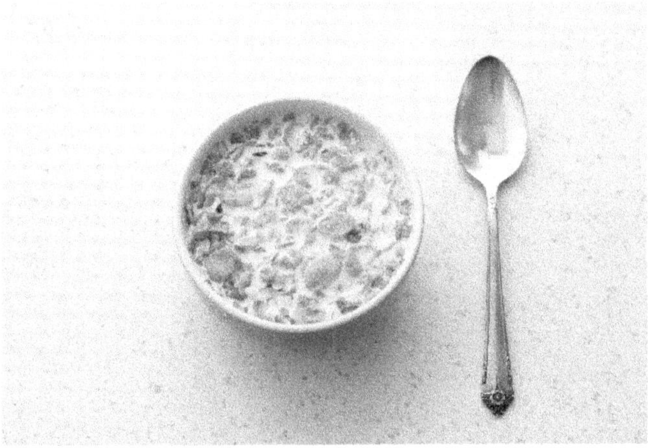

1 Tasty Oatmeal Muffins

Preparation time: 10 minutesCooking time: 20 minutes Servings: 12
Ingredients:

½ cup of hot water

½ cup of raisins

¼ cup of ground flaxseed
2 cups of rolled oats

¼ teaspoon of sea salt

½ cup of walnuts

¼ teaspoon of baking soda1 banana
2 tablespoons of cinnamon

¼ cup of maple syrupDirections:
Whisk the flaxseed with water and allow the mixture to sit for about 5 minutes.

In a food processor, blend all the ingredients along with the flaxseed mix. Blend everything for 30 seconds, but do not create a smooth substance. To create rough-textured cookies, you need to have a semi-coarse batter.

Put the batter in cupcake liners and place them in a muffin tin. As this is an oil-free recipe, you will need cupcake liners. Bake everything for about 20 minutes at 350 degrees.

Enjoy the freshly-made cookies with a glass of warm milk. Nutrition: Calories: 133, Fats 2 g, Carbohydrates 27 g, Protein 3 g

2 Omelet with Chickpea Flour

Preparation time: 10 minutesCooking time: 20 minutes Serving: 1
Ingredients:

½ teaspoon, onion powder

¼ teaspoon, black pepper1 cup, chickpea flour
½ teaspoon, garlic powder

½ teaspoon, baking soda

¼ teaspoon, white pepper1/3 cup, nutritional yeast
3 finely chopped green onions 4 ounces, sautéed mushroomsDirections:
In a small bowl, mix the onion powder, white pepper, chickpea flour, garlic powder, black and white pepper, baking soda, and nutritional yeast.

Add 1 cup of water and create a smooth batter.

On medium heat, put a frying pan and add the batter just like the way you would cook pancakes.

On the batter, sprinkle some green onion and mushrooms. Flip the omelet and cook evenly on both sides. Onceothsidesrecooked,servetheomeletwithspinach, tomatoes, hot sauce, and salsa.

Nutrition: Calories: 150, Fats 1.9 g, Carbohydrates 24.4 g, Proteins

10.2 g

3 White Sandwich Bread

Preparation: 10 minutesCooking: 20 minutes Servings: 16
Ingredients:

1 cup warm water

2 tablespoons active dry yeast4 tablespoons oil
2 ½ teaspoons salt

2 tablespoons raw sugar or 4 tablespoons maple syrup /agavenectar

1 cup warm almond milk or any other nondairy milk of your choice6 cups all-purpose flour
Directions:

Add warm water, yeast and sugar into a bowl and stir. Set aside for 5 minutes or until lots of tiny bubbles are formed, sort of frothy.

Add flour and salt into a mixing bowl and stir. Pour the oil, yeast mix and milk and mix into dough. If the dough is too hard, add a little water, a tablespoon at a time and mix well each time. If the dough is too sticky, add more flour, a tablespoon at a time. Knead the dough for 8 minutes until soft and supple. You can use your hands or use the dough hook attachment of the stand mixer.

Now spray some water on top of the dough. Keep the bowl covered with a towel. Let it rest until it doubles in size. Remove the dough from the bowl and place on your countertop. Punch the dough.Line a loaf pan with parchment paper. You can also grease with ome oil if you prefer. You can use 2 smaller loaf pans if you want to make smaller loaves, like I did.Place the dough in the loaf pan. Now spray some more water on top of the dough. Keep the loaf pan covered with a towel. Let it rest until the dough doubles in size.Bake in a preheated oven at 370° F for about 40 – 50 minutes or a toothpick when inserted in the center of the bread comes out without any particles stuck on it.Let it cool to room temperature.

Cut into 16 equal slices and use as required. Store in a breadbox at room temperature. Nutrition: Calories 209, Fat 4 g, Carbohydrate 35 g, Protein 1 g

4 Mexican-Spiced Tofu Scramble

Preparation time: 13 mCooking time: 10 m Ingredients:

1 tbsp. safflower oil

2 packages of extra-firm tofu, drained and pressed3 scallions, chopped
2 cloves garlic, minced

1 red bell pepper, chopped

½ tsp. ground cumin

½ tsp. Mexican chile powder

½ tsp. ground coriander

½ tsp. paprika

½ tsp. garlic powder

½ tsp. dried oregano

1 tsp. black salt

2 tbsp. nutritional yeast (optional)1/2 tsp. turmeric
2 tbsp. fresh cilantro, chopped

2 tbsp. ground flaxseed (optional)1-4 oz. can green chiles
1 cup of water

1-15 oz. can black beans, drained and rinsedDirections:
Heat a large frying pan over moderate heat. Add the oil and cook the chives, peppers, and garlic for about 3 minutes until tender. Breakthe tofu into large pieces and add them to the pan. Throw it away so that it is covered with aromatics and let it sit until it is golden before playing it. When browning after about 5 minutes, stir in the tofu to brown it on all sides.

While the tofu is browning, mix the spices in a small bowl or cup. Increase or reduce the amount depending on how you like spicy foods. Nutritional yeast and flax seeds are optional additions, but healthy if you have them. Add the spice blend to the pan and mix thetofu to evenly distribute the spices. Add 1 cup of water into the pan and stir. This helps the spices to distribute evenly and moistens the dispute. The water will cook.

Mix the green peppers and black beans in the tofu race. Cook for about 5 minutes until all the ingredients are hot. Mix the coriander. Serve hot.

Nutrition: Carbs: 91 g Calories: 1,113 Fat: 49 gSodium: 670 mg

Protein: 83 g Sugar: 9 g

5 Chocolate PB Smoothie

Preparation time: 5 minutesCooking time: 0 minutes Servings: 4
Ingredients1 banana
¼ cup rolled oats, or 1 scoop plant protein powder

1 tablespoon flaxseed, or chia seeds

1 tablespoon unsweetened cocoa powder

1 tablespoon peanut butter, or almond or sunflower seed butter 1 tablespoon maple syrup (optional)
1 cup alfalfa sprouts, or spinach, chopped (optional)

½ cup non-dairy milk (optional)1 cup water

Optional

1 teaspoon maca powder1 teaspoon cocoa nibs Directions
Purée everything in a blender until smooth, adding more water (or non-dairy milk) if needed. Add bonus boosters, as desired. Purée until blended.

Nutrition: calories: 474; protein: 13g; total fat: 16g; carbohydrates: 79g; fiber: 18g

6 Orange French Toast

Preparation time: 15 minutesCooking time: 10 minutes Servings: 4
Ingredients

3 very ripe bananas

1 cup unsweetened nondairy milkZest and juice of 1 orange
1 teaspoon ground cinnamon

¼ Teaspoon grated nutmeg4 slices french bread
1 tablespoon coconut oil

Directions

In a blender, combine the bananas, almond milk, orange juice and zest, cinnamon, and nutmeg and blend until smooth. Pour the mixture into a 9-by-13-inch baking dish. Soak the bread in the mixture for 5 minutes on each side.

While the bread soaks, heat a griddle or sauté pan over medium- high heat. Melt the coconut oil in the pan and swirl to coat. Cook the bread slices until golden brown on both sides, about 5 minutes each. Serve immediately.

7 Oatmeal Raisin Breakfast Cookie

Preparation: 5 minutesCooking: 15 minutes Servings: 2 cookies

Ingredients
½ Cup rolled oats 1 tablespoon whole-grain flour

½ Teaspoon baking powder to 2 tablespoons brown sugar

½ Teaspoon pumpkin pie spice or ground cinnamon (optional)

¼ Cup unsweetened applesauce, plus more as needed

1 tablespoons raisins, dried cranberries, or vegan chocolate chips
Directions
In a medium bowl, stir together the oats, flour, baking powder, sugar,

and pumpkin pie spice (if using). Stir in the applesauce until thoroughly combined. Add another 1 to 2 tablespoons of applesauce if the mixture looks too dry (this will depend on the type of oatsused).

Shape the mixture into 2 cookies. Put them on a microwave-safe plate and heat on high power for 90 seconds. Alternatively, bake ona small tray in a 350°f oven or toaster oven for 15 minutes. Let cool slightly before eating.

Nutrition (2 cookies): calories: 175; protein: 74g; total fat: 2g; saturated fat:0g; carbohydrates: 39g; fiber: 4g

8 Breakfast Blueberry Muffins

Preparation Time: 15 minutesCooking Time: 25 minutes Servings: 12
Ingredients:

Cooking spray

1 ½ cups rolled oats

¼ teaspoon baking soda1 teaspoon baking powder
½ cup unsweetened applesauce

⅓ cup packed light brown sugar

¼ teaspoon salt

3 tablespoons vegetable oil3 tablespoons water
1 tablespoon flax meal

1 teaspoon vanilla extract

¾ cup blueberries, sliced in halfDirections:
Preheat your oven to 350 degrees F.

Spray your muffin pan with oil. Add the oats in a food processor. Pulse until ground.

Stir in the rest of the ingredients except blueberries.Pulse until smooth.
Pour the batter into the muffin pan.

Top with the blueberries.

Bake in the oven for 25 minutes.Store in a glass jar with lid.

a) Nutrition:
b) Calories: 106
c) fat: 4.6g
d) Saturated fat: 0.4g
e) Sodium:118mg
f) Potassium: 66mg Carbohydrates: 15.5g
g) Fiber: 1.5g Sugar: 8gProtein: 1.5g

9 **Oatmeal with Pears**

Preparation: 15 minutesCooking: 15 minutes Serving: 1
Ingredients:

¼ cup roll ed oats ¼ cup pear, sliced

1/8 teaspoon ground ginger 1/8 teaspoon ground cinnamonDirections:
Cook the oats according to the directions in the package. Stir in pear and ginger.
Sprinkle with cinnamon. Store in a glass jar with lid.Refrigerate overnight.

Nutrition: Calories: 108 fat: 2g Saturated fat: 0.1g Sodium: 5mg Potassium: 71mg Carbohydrates: 21g Fiber: 3g Sugar: 4g Protein: 3g

10 Almond Chia Pudding

Preparation time: 10 minutesCooking time: 0 minutes Servings: 2
Ingredients:

3 tablespoons almond butter 2 tablespoons maple syrup 1 cup almond milk
¼ cup plus 1 tablespoon chia seedsDirections:
In a sealable container, add everything and mix well.Seal the container and refrigerate overnight.
Serve with a splash of almond milk.

Nutrition: Calories 212 Total Fat 11.8 g Saturated Fat 2.2 g Cholesterol 23mg Sodium 321 mg Total Carbs 14.6 g Fibers 4.4 g Sugar 8 g Protein 7.3g

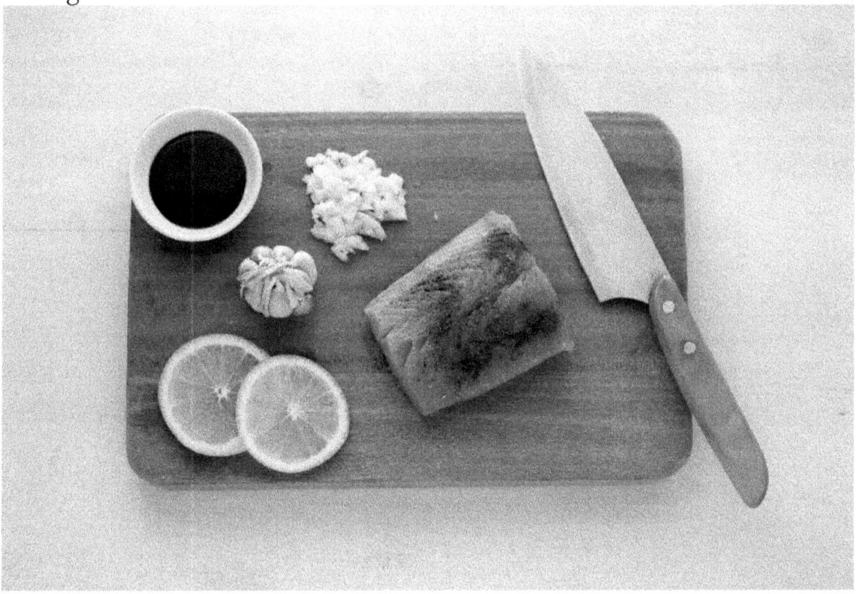

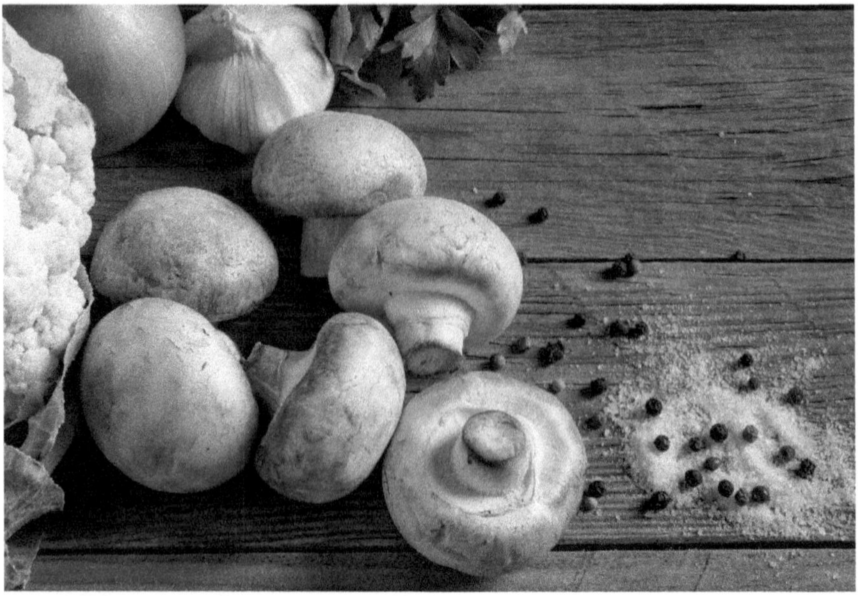

Soups, Salads, and Sides

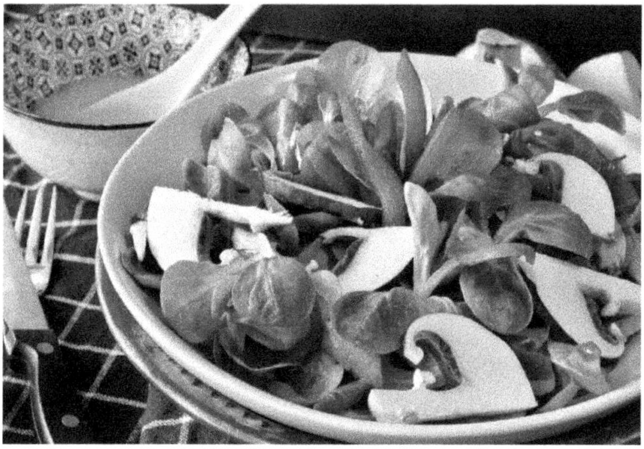

11 Spinach Soup with Dill and Basil

Preparation: 10 minutesCooking: 25 minutes Servings: 8
Ingredients:

1 pound peeled and diced potatoes1 tablespoon minced garlic 1 teaspoon dry mustard

6 cups vegetable broth

20 ounces chopped frozen spinach2 cups chopped onion
1 ½ tablespoons salt ½ cup minced dill1 cup basil
½ teaspoon ground black pepper

Directions:

Whisk onion, garlic, potatoes, broth, mustard, and salt in a pand cook it over medium flame. When it starts boiling, low down the heat and cover it with the lid and cook for 20 minutes. Add the remaining ingredients in it and blend it and cook it for few more minutes and serve it.

Nutrition: Carbohydrates 12g, protein 13g, fats 1g, calories 165.

12 Coconut Watercress Soup

Preparation time: 10 minutesCooking time: 20 minutes Servings: 4
Ingredients:

1 teaspoon coconut oil1 onion, diced
¾ cup coconut milk

Directions:

Preparing the ingredients.

Melt the coconut oil in a large pot over medium-high heat. Add the onion and cook until soft, about 5 minutes, then add the peas andthe water. Bring to a boil, then lower the heat and add the watercress, mint, salt, and pepper.

Cover and simmer for 5 minutes. Stir in the coconut milk, and purée the soup until smooth in a blender or with an immersion blender.

Try this soup with any other fresh, leafy green—anything from spinach to collard greens to arugula to swiss chard.

Nutrition: calories: 178; protein: 6g; total fat: 10g; carbohydrates: 18g; fiber: 5g

13 Roasted Red Pepper and Butternut Squash Soup

Preparation time: 10 minutesCooking time: 45 minutes Servings: 6
Ingredients:

1 small butternut squash1 tablespoon olive oil

1 teaspoon sea salt

2 red bell peppers1 yellow onion

1 head garlic

2 cups water, or vegetable brothZest and juice of 1 lime

1 to 2 tablespoons tahini

Pinch cayenne pepper

½ teaspoon ground coriander

½ teaspoon ground cumin Toasted squash seeds (optional)Directions:
Preparing the ingredients.Preheat the oven to 350°f.

Prepare the squash for roasting by cutting it in half lengthwise, scooping out the seeds, and poking some holes in the flesh with a fork. Reserve the seeds if desired.

Rub a small amount of oil over the flesh and skin, then rub with a bit of sea salt and put the halves skin-side down in a large baking dish. Put it in the oven while you prepare the rest of the vegetables.

Prepare the peppers the exact same way, except they do not need to be poked.

Slice the onion in half and rub oil on the exposed faces. Slice the top off the head of garlic and rub oil on the exposed flesh.

After the squash has cooked for 20 minutes, add the peppers, onion, and garlic, and roast for another 20 minutes. Optionally, you can toast the squash seeds by putting them in the oven in a separate baking dish 10 to 15 minutes before the vegetables are finished.

Keep a close eye on them. When the vegetables are cooked, take them out and let them cool before handling them. The squash will bevery soft when poked with a fork.

Scoop the flesh out of the squash skin into a large pot (if you havean immersion blender) or into a blender.

Chop the pepper roughly, remove the onion skin and chop the onion roughly, and squeeze the garlic cloves out of the head, all into thepot or blender. Add the water, the lime zest and juice, and the tahini. Purée the soup, adding more water if you like, to your desired consistency. Season with the salt, cayenne, coriander, and cumin. Serve garnished with toasted squash seeds (if using).

Nutrition: calories: 156; protein: 4g; total fat: 7g; saturated fat: 11g; carbohydrates: 22g; fiber: 5g

Entrées

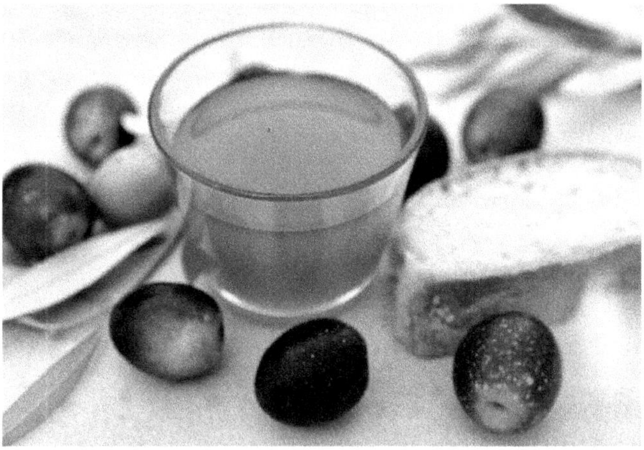

14 Black Bean Dip

Preparation time: 1 hour and 30 minutesCooking time: 1 hour
Servings: 10Ingredients:

2 15-ounce cans black beans, rinsed and drained 1 jalapeno pepper, seeded and minced

½ of a red bell pepper, seeded and diced

½ of a yellow bell pepper, seeded and diced

½ of s small red onion, diced

1 cup fresh cilantro, finely choppedZest of 1 lime
Juice of 1 lime

1 10-ounce can Ro*tel, drained

½ teaspoon Kosher salt

¼ teaspoon ground black pepperDirections:
In a large bowl, combine the garlic, green onions, beans, jalapeno,red and yellow bell pepper, onion, cilantro and mix together well.

Add the lime zest and juice, Ro-tel, salt and pepper and mix. Adjust seasoning to your own taste.

Refrigerate for at one hour, minimum, before serving, so the flavors have time to blend. Serve with wheat tortilla slices that have been crisped in the oven or with wheat or sesame crackers.

15 Cannellini Bean Cashew Dip

Preparation time: 1 hourCooking time: 1 hour Servings: 8
Ingredients:

1 15-ounce can cannellini beans, rinsed and drained

½ cup raw cashews

1 clove garlic, smashed

2 tablespoons diced, red bell pepper

½ teaspoon sea salt

¼ teaspoon cayenne pepper4 teaspoons lemon juice
2 tablespoons water

Dill sprigs or weed for garnishDirections:
Place the beans, cashews, garlic and bell pepper in the food processor and pulse several times to break it up.

Add the salt, cayenne, lemon juice and water and process until smooth.

Scrape into a bowl, cover and refrigerate for at least an hour before serving.

Garnish with fresh dill and serve with vegetables, crackers or pita chips.

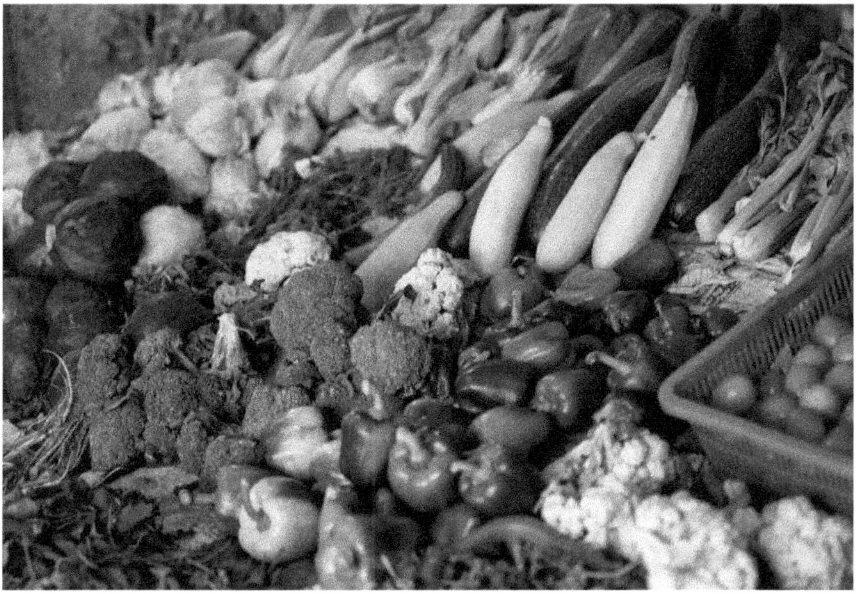

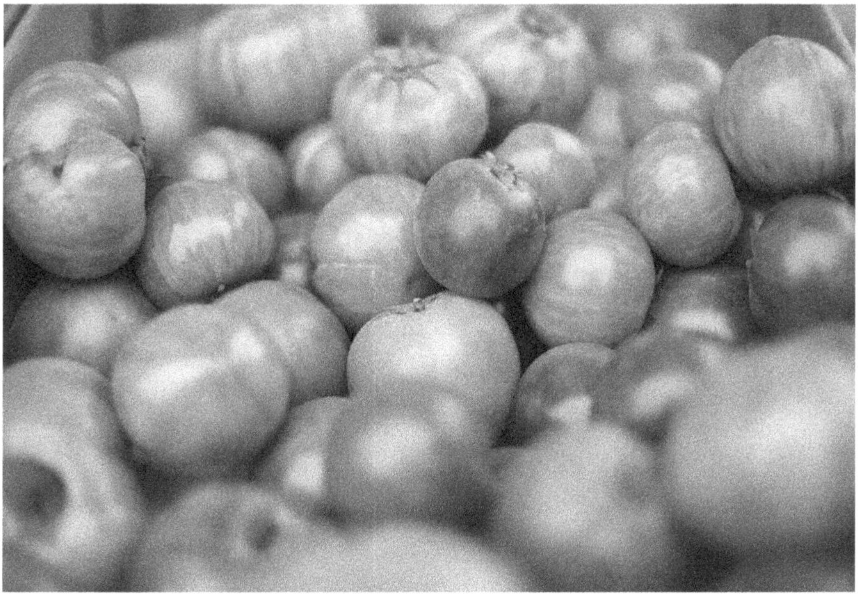

Smoothies and Beverages

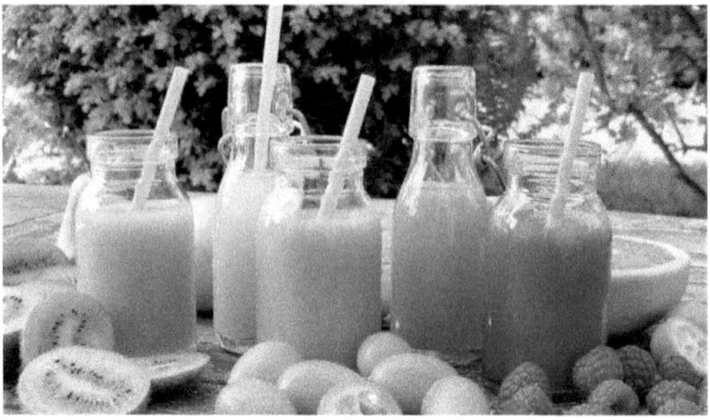

16 Fruity Smoothie

Preparation Time: 10 MinutesCooking time: 0 minute Servings: 1
Ingredients:

¾ cup soy yogurt

½ cup pineapple juice

1 cup pineapple chunks 1 cup raspberries, sliced1 cup blueberries, sliced
Direction:

Process the ingredients in a blender.Chill before serving.
Nutrition: Calories 279, Total Fat 2 g, Saturated Fat 0 g Cholesterol 4 mg, Sodium 149 mg, Total Carbohydrate 56 g Dietary Fiber 7 g, Protein 12 g, Total Sugars 46 g Potassium 719 mg

17 Energizing Ginger Detox Tonic

Preparation time: 15 minutesCooking time: 10 minutes Servings: 2
Ingredients:

1/2 teaspoon of grated ginger, fresh1 small lemon slice
1/8 teaspoon of cayenne pepper

1/8 teaspoon of ground turmeric 1/8 teaspoon of ground cinnamon 1 teaspoon of maple syrup
1 teaspoon of apple cider vinegar2 cups of boiling water Directions:
Pour the boiling water into a small saucepan, add and stir the ginger, then let it rest for 8 to 10 minutes, before covering the pan.

Pass the mixture through a strainer and into the liquid, add the cayenne pepper, turmeric, cinnamon and stir properly.

Add the maple syrup, vinegar, and lemon slice.

Add and stir an infused lemon and serve immediately.

Nutrition: Calories:80 Cal, Carbohydrates:0g, Protein:0g, Fats:0g,Fiber:0g.

18 Warm Spiced Lemon Drink

Preparation time: 2 hours and 10 minutesCooking time: 2 hours
Servings: 12

Ingredients:

1 cinnamon stick, about 3 inches long1/2 teaspoon of whole cloves
2 cups of coconut sugar

4 fluid of ounce pineapple juice

1/2 cup and 2 tablespoons of lemon juice12 fluid ounce of orange juice
2 1/2 quarts of water

Directions:

Pour water into a 6-quarts slow cooker and stir the sugar and lemonjuice properly.

Wrap the cinnamon, the whole cloves in cheesecloth and tie its corners with string.

Immerse this cheesecloth bag in the liquid present in the slow cookerand cover it with the lid.

Then plug in the slow cooker and let it cook on high heat setting for 2 hours or until it is heated thoroughly.

When done, discard the cheesecloth bag and serve the drink hot orcold.
Nutrition: Calories:15 Cal, Carbohydrates:3.2g,Pro

19 Chocolate Smoothie

Preparation Time: 5 min.Cooking Time: 5 min.
Servings: 2

Ingredients:

¼ c. almond butter

¼ c. cocoa powder, unsweetened

½ c. coconut milk, canned

1 c. almond milk, unsweetenedDirections:
Before making the smoothie, freeze the almond milk into cubesusing an ice cube tray. This would take a few hours, so prepare it ahead.

Blend everything using your preferred machine until it reaches your desired thickness.

Serve immediately and enjoy!

Nutrition: Calories: 147 | Carbohydrates: 8.2 g | Proteins: 4 g | Fats: 13.4 g

20 . Chocolate Mint Smoothie

Preparation Time: 5 min.Cooking Time: 5 min.
Serving: 1

Ingredients:

2 tbsp. sweetener of your choice2 drops mint extract
1 tbsp. cocoa powder

½ avocado, medium

¼ c. coconut milk

1 c. almond milk, unsweetenedDirections:
In a high-speed blender, add all the ingredients and blend untilsmooth.

Add two to four ice cubes and blend.Serve immediately and enjoy!
Nutrition: Calories: 401 | Carbohydrates: 6.3 g | Proteins: 5 g | Fats: 40.3 g

21 Cinnamon Roll Smoothie

Preparation: 2 min.Cooking: 2 min. Serving: 1

Ingredients:

1 t. cinnamon 1 scoop vanilla protein powder

½ c. of the following: almond milk, unsweetened

- coconut milk Sweetener of your choiceDirections:

In a high-speed blender, add all the ingredients and blend.Add two to four ice cubes and blend until smooth.
Serve immediately and enjoy!

Nutrition: Calories: 507 | Carbohydrates: 17 g | Proteins: 33.3 g | Fats: 34.9 g

22 Coconut Smoothie

Preparation: 2 min.Cooking: 2 min.Servings: 2Ingredients:
1 t. chia seeds 1/8 c. almonds, soaked1 c. coconut milk
1 avocado

Directions:

In a high-speed blender, add all the ingredients and blend until smooth.Add your desired number of ice cubes, depending on your favored consistency, of course, and blend again. Serve immediately and enjoy!

Nutrition: Calories: 584 | Carbohydrates: 22.5 g | Proteins: 8.3 g | Fats: 55.5g

Snacks and Desserts

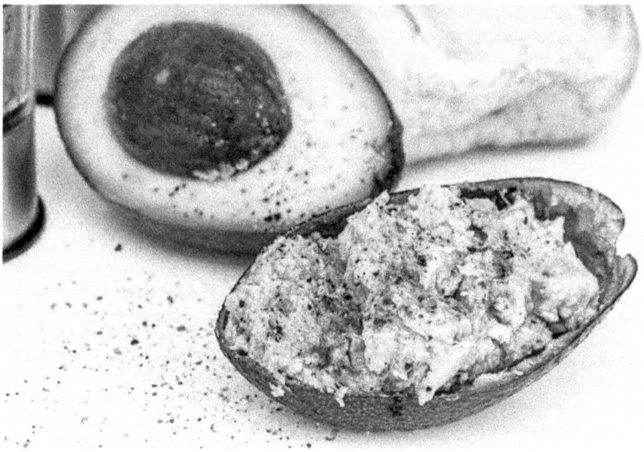

23 Mango And Banana Shake

Preparation time: 10 minsCooking time: 0 mins Servings: 2
Ingredients:

1 Banana, Sliced And Frozen1 Cup Frozen Mango Chunks1 Cup Almond Milk

1 Tbsp. Maple Syrup1 Tsp Lime Juice
2-4 Raspberries For Topping

Mango Slice For ToppingDirections
In blender, pulse banana, mango with milk, maple syrup, lime juice until smooth but still thick

Add more liquid if needed.Pour shake into 2 bowls.
Top with berries and mango slice.

Enjoy!

Nutrition: Protein: 5% 8 kcal Fat: 11% 18 kcal Carbohydrates: 85% 140 kcal

24 Avocado Toast With Flaxseeds

Preparation time: 5 mins.Cooking time: 0 mins Servings: 3
Ingredients:

3 slice of whole grain bread1 large avocado, ripe
¼ cup chopped parsley

1 tbsp. flax seeds

1 tbsp. sesame seeds1 tbsp. lime juice Directions:
First, toast your piece of bread.Remove the avocado seed.
Slice half avocado and mash half avocado with fork in bowl. Spread mashed avocado on 2 toasted bread.
Place avocado slice on 1 toast.

Top with flax seeds and sesame seeds. Drizzle lime juice and chopped parsley on top.Serve and enjoy!
Nutrition: Protein: 12% 31 kcal Fat: 49% 124 kcal Carbohydrates:

39% 98 kcal

25 Avocado Hummus

Preparation time: 10 minsCooking time:
Servings: 4

Ingredients

2 Ripe Avocados

½ Cup Coconut Cream

¼ Cup Sesame Paste

½ Lemon Juice

1 Tsp. Clove, Pressed

½ Tsp Ground Cumin

½ Tsp Salt

¼ Tsp Ground Black PepperDirections
Cut the avocado lengthways and remove seed from the fruit.

Put all ingredients in a blender or food processor and mix untilthoroughly smooth.

Add more cream, lemon juice or water if you want to have a looser texture.

Adjust seasonings as needed.Serve with naan and enjoy.
Nutrition: Protein: 6% 21 kcal Fat: 79% 289 kcal Carbohydrates:

16% 57 kcal

26 Beans with Sesame Hummus

Preparation time: 10 minutesCooking time: 0 minutes Servings: 6
Ingredients

4 Tbsp sesame oil

2 cloves garlic finely sliced

1 can (15 oz) cannellini beans, drained
4 Tbsp sesame paste

2 Tbsp lemon juice freshly squeezed1/4 tsp red pepper flakes
2 Tbsp fresh basil finely chopped

2 Tbsp fresh parsley finely choppedSea salt to taste
Directions:

Place all ingredients in your food processor.

Process until all ingredients are combined well and smooth. Transfer mixture into a bowl and refrigerate until servings.

27 Candied Honey-Coconut Peanuts

Preparation time: 15 minutesCooking time: 10 minutes Servings: 8
Ingredients

1/2 cup honey (preferably a darker honey)4 Tbsp coconut butter softened
1 tsp ground cinnamon

4 cups roasted, salted peanutsDirections
Add honey, coconut butter, and cinnamon in a microwave-safe bowl. Microwave at HIGH for about 4 to 5 minutes.
Stir in nuts; mix thoroughly to coat.

Microwave at HIGH 5 to 6 minutes or until foamy; stir after 3minutes.

Spread in a single layer on a greased tray.Refrigerated for 6 hours.
Break into small pieces and serve.

28 Choco Walnuts Fat Bombs

Preparation time: 15 minutesCooking time: 0 minutes Servings: 6 Ingredients

1/2 cup coconut butter

1/2 cup coconut oil softened

4 Tbs cocoa powder, unsweetened4 Tbs brown sugar firmly packed 1/3 cup silken tofu mashed
1 cup walnuts, roughly choppedDirections
Add coconut butter and coconut oil into a microwave dish; melt it for 10-15 seconds.

Add in cocoa powder and whisk well.

Pour mixture into a blender with brown sugar and silken tofu cream; blend for 3-4 minutes.

Place silicone molds onto a sheet pan and fill halfway with chopped walnuts.

Pour the mixture over the walnuts and place it in the freezer for 6 hours.

Ready! Serve!

29 Spiced Chickpeas

Preparation Time: 45 MinutesCooking Time: 40 minutes Servings: 4
Ingredients:

Cayenne Pepper (.10 t.)Dried Oregano (.25 t.) Garlic Powder (.10 t.) Salt (to Taste)
Olive Oil (2 T.) Chickpeas (1 Can)Directions:
Start this recipe by prepping the oven to 450 and lining a baking sheet with parchment paper.

Take a mixing bowl, add in chickpeas and coat with the spices and olive oil. Once this is done, pop everything into the oven for 40 minutes.

After 40 minutes, remove the pan from the oven, allow it to cool completely and enjoy.

Nutrition: Calories: 170 Proteins: 7g Carbs: 31g Fats: 2g

Dinner Recipes

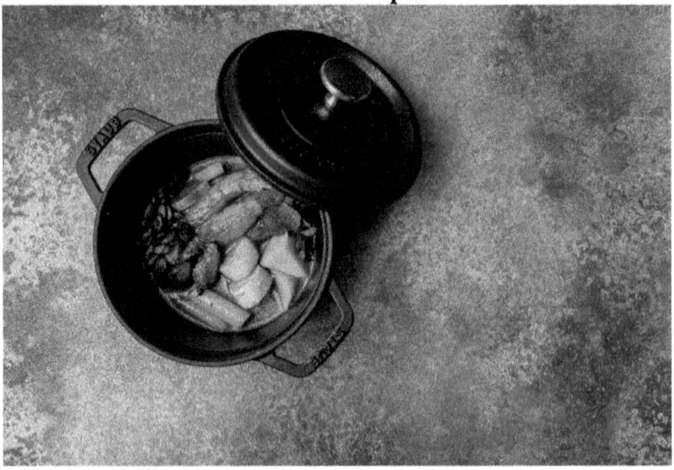

30 Mushroom Steak

Preparation Time: 30 min.Cooking Time: 1 hr.
Servings: 8

Ingredients:

1 tbsp. of the following:fresh lemon juice
olive oil, extra virgin

2 tbsp. coconut oil3 thyme sprigs
8 medium Portobello mushroomsFor Sauce:
1 ½ t. of the following:minced garlic
minced peeled fresh ginger2 tbsp. of the following: light brown sugar
mirin

½ c. low-sodium soy sauceDirections:

For the sauce, combine all the sauce ingredients, along with ¼ cup water into a little pan and simmer to cook. Cook using a medium heat until it reduces to a glaze, approximately 15 to 20 minutes, then remove from the heat.

For the mushrooms, bring the oven to 350 heat setting.

Using a skillet, melt coconut oil and olive oil, cooking the mushroomson each side for about 3 minutes.

Next, arrange the mushrooms in a single layer on a sheet for bakingand season with lemon juice, salt, and pepper.

Carefully slide into the oven and roast for 5 minutes. Let it rest for 2 minutes.

Plate and drizzle the sauce over the mushrooms.Enjoy.
Nutrition: Calories: 87 | Carbohydrates: 6.2 g | Proteins: 3 g | Fats: 6.2 g

31 Broccoli & black beans stir fry

Preparation time 60 minutesCooking time: 10 minutes Servings: 6
Ingredients:

4 cups broccoli flore ts

2 cups cooked black beans1 tablespoon sesame oil
4 teaspoons sesame seeds 2 cloves garlic, finely minced
2 teaspoons ginger, finely chopped A large pinch red chili flakesA pinch turmeric powderSalt to taste
Lime juice to taste (optional)

Direction:

Steam broccoli for 6 minutes. Drain and set aside.

Warm the sesame oil in a large frying pan over medium heat. Add sesame seeds, chili flakes, ginger, garlic, turmeric powder, and salt. Sauté for a couple of minutes.

Add broccoli and black beans and sauté until thoroughly heated.

Sprinkle lime juice and serve hot.

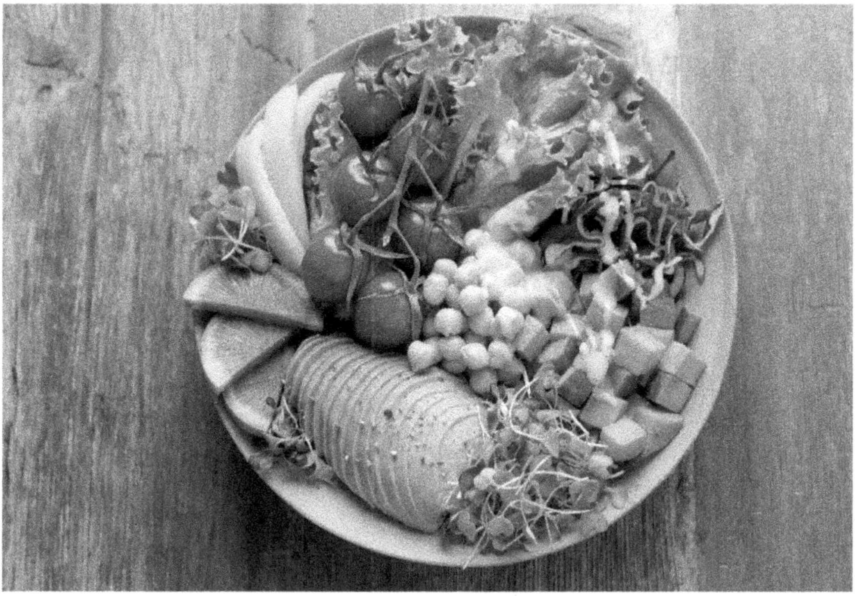

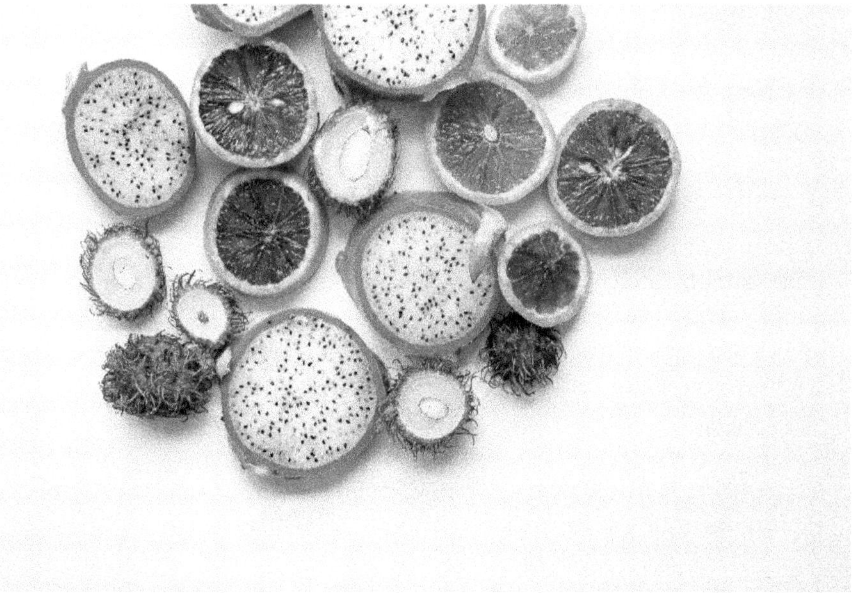

Lunch Recipes

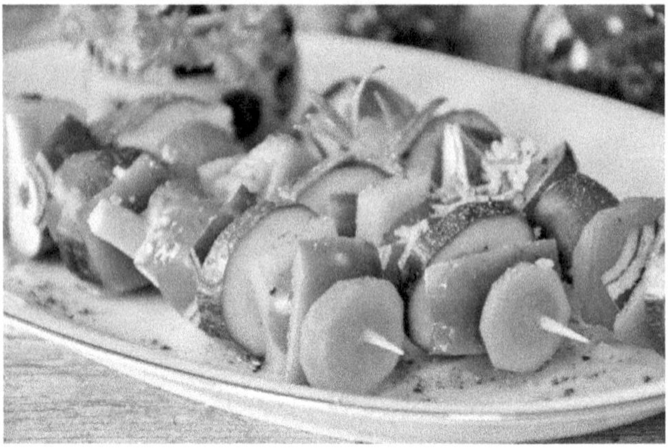

32 Teriyaki Tofu Stir-Fry

Preparation time: 10 minutesCooking Time: 20 minutes Serving: 4
Ingredients:

For the Tofu:

1 tablespoons chopped green onions2 cups asparagus
14 ounces (397 grams) tofu, firm, pressed

2 teaspoons red chili sauce1 tablespoon soy sauce
3 teaspoons olive oilFor the Sauce:
2 tablespoons minced garlic 1 ½ tablespoons rice vinegar1/2 tablespoon grated ginger2 teaspoons corn starch
1/4 cup (59 grams) coconut sugar3 tablespoons soy sauce
1 tablespoon sesame oil1/2 cup (118 ml) water
For Serving:

4 cups (946 grams) quinoa, cookedDirections:
Prepare the tofu: pat dry tofu and cut into ½-inch cubes.

Take a medium skillet pan, place it over medium-high heat, add 1 teaspoon oil and when hot, add tofu cubes in a single layer, then cook for 3 to 4 minutes until golden brown.

Transfer tofu pieces to a large bowl, add 1 teaspoon oil in the pan and repeat with the remaining tofu cubes.

Meanwhile, prepare the sauce: take a small bowl, add all of the sauce ingredients in it and whisk until combined, then set aside until required.

When all the tofu gets cooked, drizzle them with sauces and toss until coated, set aside until required.

Wipe clean the skillet pan, return it over medium-high heat, add remaining oil and when hot, add asparagus and green onions, then cook for 3 minutes until tender-crisp.

Return tofu pieces into the pan, drizzle with prepared sauce, switch heat to medium level, toss until all the ingredients are mixed, and cook for 3 to 5 minutes until the sauce starts to thicken.

When done, taste to adjust the seasoning of the sauce and then remove the pan from heat.

Distribute cooked quinoa among plates, top with tofu and vegetables, and then serve.

Nutrition: 411 Cal; 11 g Fat; 1 g Saturated Fat; 58 g Carbs; 8 g Fiber;

19 g Protein; 12 g Sugar

33 Cauliflower Latke

Preparation Time: 15 minutesCooking Time: 30 minutes Servings: 4
Ingredients:

12 oz. cauliflower rice, cooked1 egg, beaten
1/3 cup cornstarch

Salt and pepper to taste

¼ cup vegetable oil, dividedChopped onion chives Direction

Squeeze excess water from the cauliflower rice using paper towels. Place the cauliflower rice in a bowl.
Stir in the egg and cornstarch.

Season with salt and pepper.

Pour 2 tablespoons of oil into a pan over medium heat.

Add 2 to 3 tablespoons of the cauliflower mixture into the pan.Cook for 3 minutes per side or until golden.
Repeat until you've used up the rest of the batter. Garnish with chopped chives.
Nutrition: Calories: 209 Total fat: 15.2g Saturated fat: 1.4g Cholesterol: 47mg Sodium: 331mg Potassium: 21mg Carbohydrates: 13.4g Fiber: 1.9g Sugar: 2g Protein: 3.4g

34 Roasted Brussels Sprouts

Preparation Time: 30 minutesCooking Time: 20 minutes Servings: 4
Ingredients:

1 lb. Brussels sprouts, sliced in half1 shallot, chopped
1 tablespoon olive oil

Salt and pepper to taste

2 teaspoons balsamic vinegar

¼ cup pomegranate seeds

¼ cup goat cheese, crumbledDirection:
Preheat your oven to 400 degrees F.

Coat the Brussels sprouts with oil.Sprinkle with salt and pepper.
Transfer to a baking pan.

Roast in the oven for 20 minutes.Drizzle with the vinegar.
Sprinkle with the seeds and cheese before serving.

Nutrition: Calories: 117 Total fat: 5.7g Saturated fat: 1.8g Cholesterol:4mg Sodium: 216mg Potassium: 491mg Carbohydrates: 13.6g Fiber: 4.8g Sugar: 5g Protein: 5.8g

35 Vegan Chicken & Rice

Preparation Time: 15 minutes

Cooking Time: 3 hours and 30 minutesServings: 8
Ingredients:

8 Tofu thighs

Salt and pepper to taste

½ teaspoon ground coriander 2 teaspoons ground cumin 17 oz. brown rice, cooked
30 oz. black beans

1 tablespoon olive oil Pinch cayenne pepper2 cups pico de gallo
¾ cup radish, sliced thinly2 avocados, sliced Direction
Season the tofu with salt, pepper, coriander and cumin. Place in a slow cooker.
Pour in the stock.

Cook on low for 3 hours and 30 minutes.Place the tofu in a cutting board.
Shred the chicken.

Toss the tofu shreds in the cooking liquid.

Serve the rice in bowls, topped with the tofu and the rest of the ingredients.

Nutrition: Calories: 470 Total fat: 17g Saturated fat: 3g Sodium: 615mg Carbohydrates: 40g Fiber: 11g Sugar: 1g Protein: 40g

36 Quinoa Buddha Bowl

Preparation Time: 10 MinutesCooking Time: 0 minutes Servings: 1
Ingredients:

Avocado (1, Diced) Cooked Quinoa (.75 C.)Pico de Gallo (3 T.) Hummus (.25 C.)
Black Beans (.75 C.)Lime Juice (1 T.) Directions:
Before you begin this recipe, you will want to cook your quinoa ahead of time according to the directions on the package.

Once the quinoa is cooked, mix it in a bowl with the beans and the hummus. Stir everything together before squeezing in the lime juice. Finally, top the bowl off with avocado and Pico de Gallo, and lunch is served.

Nutrition: Calories: 26 Proteins: 26gCarbs: 30g Fats: 20g

37 Lettuce Hummus Wrap

Preparation Time: 5 MinutesCooking Time: 0 Minutes Servings: 4
Ingredients:

Lettuce (.50 C.)

Spinach Wraps (4)

Tomato (.50, Sliced) Carrots (.50 C., Shredded)Cucumber (.50, Diced)
Hummus (.50 C.)

Tomato (.50, Diced)

Red Bell Pepper (.50, Diced)Directions:
To make these delicious wraps, simply layout each spinach wrap andspread a layer of hummus on first.

Once the hummus is down, layer whichever vegetables you like overthe top, roll, and enjoy!

Nutrition: Calories: 25 Proteins: 2g Carbs: 6g Fats: 6g

38 Simple Curried Vegetable Rice

Preparation: 30 MinutesCooking: 10 Minutes Servings: 4
Ingredients:

Carrots (2, Chopped) Spinach (1 C., Chopped)Ginger (2 t.)
Broccoli (1, Chopped)Salt (to Taste)
Cooked Brown Rice (1 C.)

Garlic (2, Minced) Pepper (to Taste) Curry Powder (1 t.)Directions:
Before you begin cooking, you will want to take some prep time to chop up all of your vegetables beforehand. When they are cut into smaller pieces, this means they will cook faster! Once your ingredients are prepared, take out a pan and begin to heat it over a medium heat. Once warm, add in some olive oil and then sprinkle in the garlic and the ginger.Next, you will want to add in the broccoli and carrots. At this point, season with salt and pepper and cook for two minutes.

Once the vegetables are cooked to your liking, add in the cooked brown rice along with the curry powder and toss the ingredients until everything is well coated.

Finally, add in the spinach and cook for another minute or until it becomes wilted. Season with some more salt and pepper, and then your meal will be ready just like that!

Nutrition: Calories: 280 Proteins: 10g Carbs: 50g Fats: 5g

39 Mushrooms and Chard Soup

Preparation time: 10 minutesCooking time: 30 minutes Servings: 4
Ingredients:

3 cups Swiss chard, chopped6 cups vegetable stock
1 cup mushrooms, sliced2 garlic cloves, minced

1 tablespoon olive oil

2 scallions, chopped

2 tablespoons balsamic vinegar

¼ cup basil, chopped

Salt and black pepper to the taste 1 tablespoon cilantro, chopped
Directions:
Heat up a pot with the oil over medium high heat, add the scallionsand the garlic and sauté for 5 minutes.

Add the mushrooms and sauté for another 5 minutes.

Add the rest of the ingredients, toss, bring to a simmer and cook over medium heat for 20 minutes more.

Ladle the soup into bowls and serve.

Nutrition: calories 140, fat 4, fiber 2, carbs 4, protein 8

Recipes For Main Courses And Single Dishes

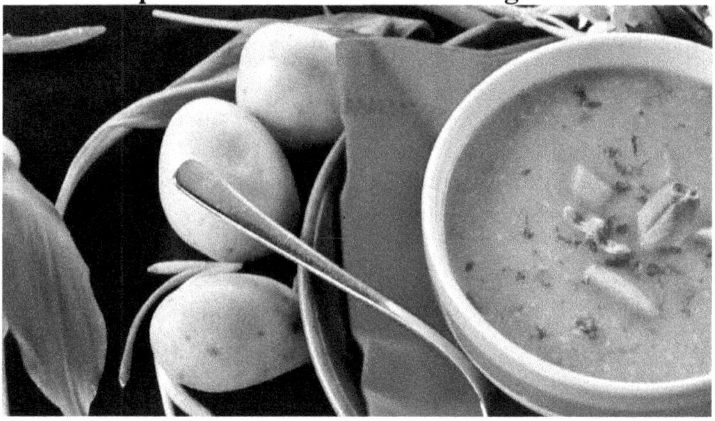

40 Noodles Alfredo with Herby Tofu

Preparation: 10 minutesCooking: 5 minutes Servings: 4
Ingredients:

2 tbsp vegetable oil

2 (14 oz.) blocks extra-firm tofu, pressed and cubed 12 ounces eggless noodles

1 tbsp dried mixed herbs

2 cups cashews, soaked overnight and drained

¾ cups unsweetened almond milk

½ cup nutritional yeast

4 garlic cloves, roasted (roasting is optional but highlyrecommended)

½ cup onion, coarsely chopped1 lemon, juiced
½ cup sun-dried tomatoes

Salt and black pepper to taste

2 tbsp chopped fresh basil leaves to garnishDirections:
Heat the vegetable oil in a large skillet over medium heat.

Season the tofu with the mixed herbs, salt, black pepper, and fry inthe oil until golden brown. Transfer to a paper-towel-lined plate and set aside. Turn the heat off.

In a blender, combine the almond milk, nutritional yeast, garlic, onion, and lemon juice. Set aside.Reheat the vegetable oil in the skillet over medium heat and sauté the noodles for 2 minutes. Stir in the sundried tomatoes and the cashew (Alfredo) sauce. Reduce the heat to low and cook for 2 more minutes.If the sauce is too thick, thin with some more almond milk to your desired thickness.

Dish the food, garnish with the basil and serve warm.

41 Lemon Couscous with Tempeh Kabobs

Preparation Time: 2 hours 15 minutesCooking Time: 2 hours
Servings: 4

Ingredients:

For the tempeh kabobs:

1 ½ cups of water

10 oz. tempeh, cut into 1-inch chunks1 red onion, cut into 1-inch chunks
1 small yellow squash, cut into 1-inch chunks

1 small green squash, cut into 1-inch chunks2 tbsp. olive oil
1 cup sugar-free barbecue sauce8 wooden skewers, soaked
For the lemon couscous:

1 ½ cups whole wheat couscous2 cups of water
Salt to taste

¼ cup chopped parsley

¼ chopped mint leaves

¼ cup chopped cilantro1 lemon, juiced
1 medium avocado, pitted, sliced and peeledDirections:

For the tempeh kabobs:

Boil the water in a medium pot over medium heat.

Once boiled, turn the heat off, and put the tempeh in it. Cover the lid and let the tempeh steam for 5 minutes (this is to remove its bitterness). Drain the tempeh after.

After, pour the barbecue sauce into a medium bowl, add the tempeh,and coat well with the sauce. Cover the bowl with plastic wrap and marinate for 2 hours.

After 2 hours, preheat a grill to 350 F.

On the skewers, alternately thread single chunks of the tempeh, onion, yellow squash, and green squash until the ingredients are exhausted.

Lightly grease the grill grates with olive oil, place the skewers on top and brush with some barbecue sauce. Cook for 3 minutes on each side while brushing with more barbecue sauce as you turn the kabobs.

Transfer to a plate for serving.For the lemon couscous:
Meanwhile, as the kabobs cooked, pour the couscous, water, and

salt into a medium bowl and steam in the microwave for 3 to 4 minutes. Remove the bowl from the microwave and allow slightcooling.

Stir in the parsley, mint leaves, cilantro, and lemon juice.

Garnish the couscous with the avocado slices and serve with the tempeh kabobs.

42 Portobello Burger with Veggie Fries

Preparation Time: 45 minutesCooking Time: 30 minutes Servings: 4
Ingredients:

For the veggie fries:

3 carrots, peeled and julienned

2 sweet potatoes, peeled and julienned1 rutabaga, peeled and julienned
2 tsp olive oil

¼ tsp paprika

Salt and black pepper to tasteFor the Portobello burgers:
1 clove garlic, minced

½ tsp salt

2 tbsp. olive oil

4 whole-wheat buns

4 Portobello mushroom caps

½ cup sliced roasted red peppers

2 tbsp. pitted Kalamata olives, chopped2 medium tomatoes, chopped
½ tsp dried oregano

¼ cup crumbled feta cheese (optional)1 tbsp. red wine vinegar
2 cups baby salad greens

½ cup hummus for servingDirections:
For the veggie fries:

Preheat the oven to 400 F.

Spread the carrots, sweet potatoes, and rutabaga on a baking sheet and season with the olive oil, paprika, salt, and black pepper. Use your hands to rub the seasoning well onto the vegetables. Bake in the oven for 20 minutes or until the vegetables soften (stir halfway).

When ready, transfer to a plate and use it for serving. For the Portobello burgers:

Meanwhile, as the vegetable roast, heat a grill pan over medium heat.

Use a spoon to crush the garlic with salt in a bowl. Stir in 1 tablespoon of the olive oil.

Brush the mushrooms on both sides with the garlic mixture and grillin the pan on both sides until tender, 8 minutes. Transfer to a plate and set aside.

Toast the buns in the pan until crispy, 2 minutes. Set aside in a plate.

In a bowl, combine the remaining ingredients except for the hummusand divide on the bottom parts of the buns.

Top with the hummus, cover the burger with the top parts of the bunsand serve with the veggie fries.

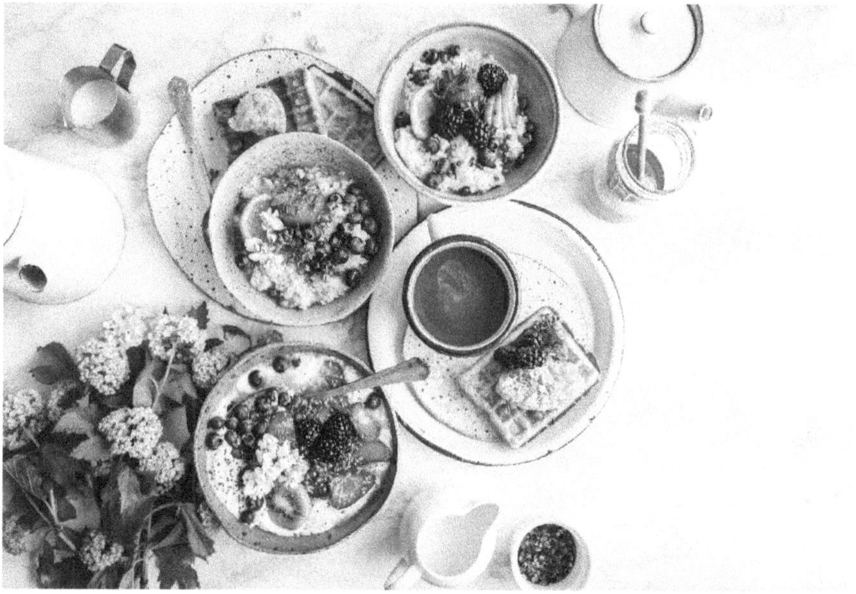

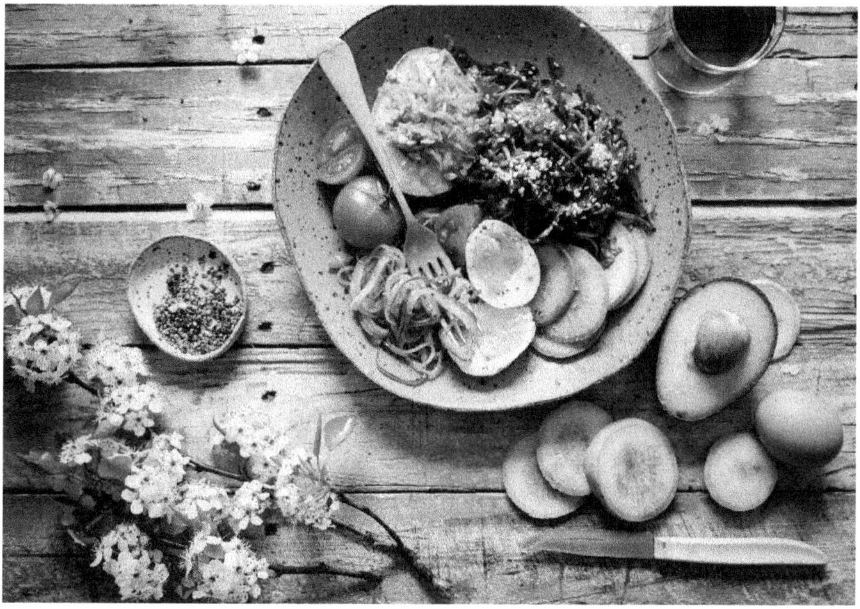

Nutrient-Packed Protein Salads

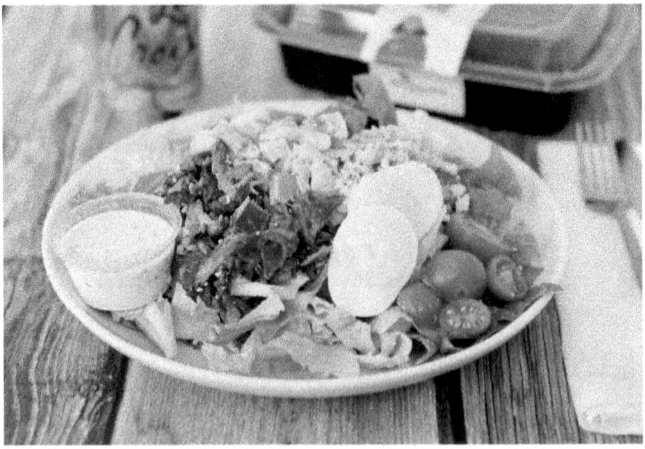

43 Grilled Halloumi Broccoli Salad

Preparation time: 15 minsCooking time: 15 mins.
Ingredient: Fresh Salad

Halloumi Cheese (about 2/3 of a packet)Half an Avocado
Baby Broccoli Quinoa (half a cup) Olive Oil (dressing).Directions:
The first thing to do is to prepare your salad. Wash and dry it well. Once the halloumi is ready, you're going to want to eat it straight away as it tends to get very rubbery as it cools off so preparing everything else beforehand makes everything easier. Prepare half anavocado by slicing it into small cubes (it'll add creaminess to your salad which is why I tend to only use olive oil as my dressing).

In a pot, add some water to boil (with a pinch of salt) for the baby broccoli. I like mine fairly crunchy so 2-3 minutes was enough. Once your salad and avocado are done and your broccoli is cooking, start with your quinoa. Put half a cup of quinoa into a small pot, add about one cup of water and leave to boil (salt isn't necessary here becauseof the saltiness of the halloumi cheese) on a medium flame.

As your broccoli is cooking, prepare your grill pan for the halloumi cheese. On a medium flame, add a few drops of olive oil and leave it to heat up. Slice the halloumi into about centimetre thick pieces, thenadd to the grill pan. Your broccoli should be ready by now so add those too. For a golden-brown colour, I grilled my halloumi and broccoli for about 6 minutes, making sure to flip the cheese over to cook it evenly.

Don't forget to check on the quinoa. It should be ready once the water is gone (about 7-8 minutes), but taste to be sure (it should have a somewhat crunchy texture). Once the halloumi, broccoli, and quinoa are ready, throw everything into your salad bowl and mix well. Season with some olive oil and serve while the halloumi is hot.

Flavour Boosters (Fish Glazes, Meat Rubs & Fish Rubs)

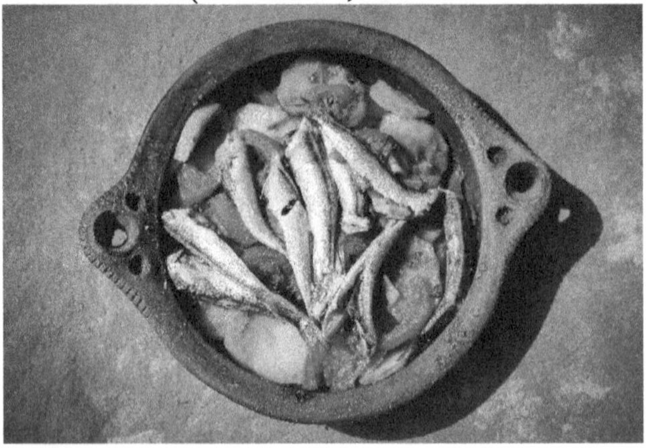

44 Classic Honey Mustard Fish Glaze

Complement your choice of fish including salmon by infusing it with succulent flavors and a perfectly glazed look by this classic honey mustard glaze.

Honey and mustard are versatile and fun, as they let you experiment endlessly and discover something new every time.

Preparation Time: 5 min.Cooking Time: 5 min.
Servings: 1/2 cup/4 oz.Ingredients:
Dijon mustard - 2 tsp.

Soy sauce (low sodium) - 4 tbsp.Honey - 6 tbsp.
Lime juice - 2 tsp.Directions:
To make the honey mustard fish glaze, combine the mustard, soy sauce, lime juice, and honey in your medium-sized bowl. Gently blend the ingredients.

Then, add the mixture into your medium-sized saucepan. Let the mixture simmer gradually for about 2 minutes.

Now, take your favorite cooked/grilled/baked salmon or any other fish variety. Gently spread or pour the prepared glaze over the fish/salmon. Allow a few minutes for the glaze to set in. Enjoy the mustard glazed fish meal!

45 Maple Syrup Spiced Fish Glaze

Give your parties and occasions a rich and classic upgrade with this maple syrup glaze. Nutmeg, combined with sharp flavors of cinnamon, makes this yummy fish glaze perfect to prepare holiday orseasonal meals.

Preparation Time: 5 min.Cooking Time: 5 min.
Servings: 1 cup/8 oz.

Ingredients:

Apple cider vinegar - 1/2 cupApple cider - 1/2 cup
Olive oil - 1 tbs. Brown sugar - 2 tbs.Maple syrup - 1 tbs.Cinnamon - 2 tsp.
Salt - 1 tsp.

Nutmeg - 1 tsp.

Onion powder - 1/2 tsp.

Directions:

To make the maple syrup glaze, combine all m
the ingredients.

Now, take your favorite cooked/grilled/baked baked salmon or any other fish variety. Gently spread or pour the prepared glaze over the cuts. Allow a few minutes for the glaze to set in. Enjoy the maple syrup-glazed fish meal!

46 Oregano Cumin Tilapia Rub

This rub is a family-friendly way to savor an earthy, mild combination of spices in your favorite fish meals. The rub includes mild flavors, suitable even for children. Apart from Tilapia, it is also perfect for varieties of fish including salmon. Enjoy with mashed potatoes!

Preparation Time: 5 min.Cooking Time: 5 min.
Servings: 4-5 tsp.Ingredients:
Light brown sugar – 1 1/2 tsp.

Paprika – 1 1/2 tsp. Dried oregano - 1 tsp.Cumin - 1/2 tsp. Garlic powder - 3/4 tsp. Cayenne pepper - 1/4 tsp.Salt - 1 tsp. Directions:

Mix in all mentioned ingredients in your mixing bowl to make the cumin tilapia rub. Gently mix all the ingredients using spatula or spoon to form an aromatic rub mixture.

Now, take your choice of fish and place it on a firm surface. Brush or rub the freshly made rub on it; pat gently for the rub to stick on the surface. Turn it and repeat to spice up its other side.

Let your fish cuts adequately season for more rich flavors for some time in your refrigerator.

*Do not let your fish season for more than 2 hours (but not less than30 minutes).

Take it out, as it is ready to be cooked or grilled!

47 Spicy Sumac Rub

This special spicy rub perfectly complements different choices of fish; it adds up extra flavors to your fish-based meals. I mean, no one likes to compromise on the mild, mouth-watering taste of Tilapia.

Preparation Time: 5 min.Cooking Time: 5 min.
Servings: 2-3 tsp.Ingredients:
Dried thyme - 1/2 tsp. Powdered sumac - 1/2 tsp.
Any variety of Creole seasoning - 1/2 tsp.Onion powder - 1/4 tsp. Garlic powder - 1/4 tsp.

Salt - 1/4 tsp. Directions:

Mix all mentioned ingredients in your mixing bowl to make the spicy

sumac rub. Gently mix all ingredients using spatula or spoon to forman aromatic rub mixture.

Now, take your choice of fish and place it on a firm surface. Brush or rub the freshly made rub on it; pat gently for the rub to stick onto the surface. Turn it and repeat to spice up its other side.

Let your fish cuts adequately season for more rich flavors for some time in your refrigerator.

*Do not let your fish season for more than 2 hours (but not less than 30 minutes).

Take it out, as it is ready to be cooked or grilled!

48 Lemon Pepper Coriander Rub

This intelligently created pepper coriander rub provides hints of tartness along with mild spiciness with inclusion of chili powder. A great choice of rub to flavor-up your weekend nights as well as any night you wish to make special.

Partner your fish meals prepared with this special rub with red wine for a truly refreshing meal time.

Preparation Time: 5 min.Cooking Time: 5 min.
Servings: ½ cup + 3 tsp.Ingredients:
Chili powder - 1 tbsp.

Lemon pepper seasoning - ¼ cupGround cumin - 1 tbsp.
Light brown sugar, firmly packed - 1 ½ tsp.Ground coriander - 1 tbsp.
Kosher salt - ½ tsp.

Ground black pepper - 1 ¼ tsp.Red pepper flakes - ½ tsp.
Directions:

Mix in all mentioned ingredients in your mixing bowl to make the lemon coriander rub. Gently mix all the ingredients using spatula or spoon to form an aromatic rub mixture.

Now, take your choice of fish and place it on a firm surface. Brush or rub the freshly made rub on it; pat gently for the rub onto stick on thesurface. Turn it and repeat to spice up its other side.

Let your fish cuts adequately season for more rich flavors for some time in your refrigerator.

*Do not let your fish season for more than 2 hours (but not less than 30 minutes).

Take it out, as it is ready to be cooked or grilled!

Sauce Recipes

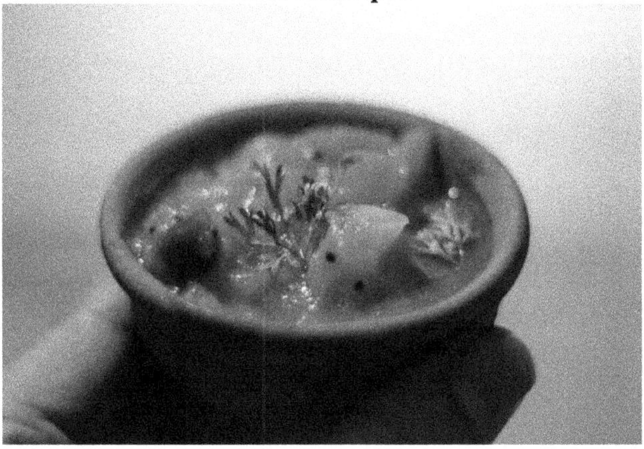

49 Runner Recovery Bites

Preparation time: 10 minutesCooking time: 10 minutes Servings: 12
Ingredients:

1/4 cup pumpkin seeds, soaked for 1 hour1/3 cup oats
1/4 cup sunflower seeds, soaked for 1 hour5 dates
1 teaspoon maca powder1 tablespoon goji berries
1 teaspoon coconut, shredded and unsweetened 1 tablespoon coconut water 1 teaspoon vanilla extract

1 tablespoon protein powder 1 tablespoon maple syrup 1/4 cup hemp seeds A pinch sea saltDirections:
Drain sunflower and pumpkin seeds and add to a blender. Blend until a paste forms. Add dates and blend to mix. Add the remaining ingredients except hemp seeds and blend until a dough forms.

Roll 1 tablespoon dough into balls with hands. Roll the ball in hemp seeds until covered.

Transfer the prepared balls to a plate and freeze until firm.Serve and enjoy.

50 High Protein Vegan Cheesy Sauce

Preparation time: 10 minutes Cooking time: 10 minutes Servings: 2 cups
Ingredients:
1 1/4 cups unsweetened plant-based milk

1 block tofu

1 teaspoon onion powder 2 teaspoon garlic powder 1/2 cup nutritional yeast 1/4 teaspoon turmeric 3/4 teaspoon salt Directions:
Add all ingredients to a blender and blend until smooth. Combine well. Add more milk as desired.

Refrigerate for 24 hours.Serve and enjoy.

Plant Based Diet Recipes 2021

A Collection of Healthy Plant-Based Recipes for Losing Weight and Healthy Eating

Frank Smith

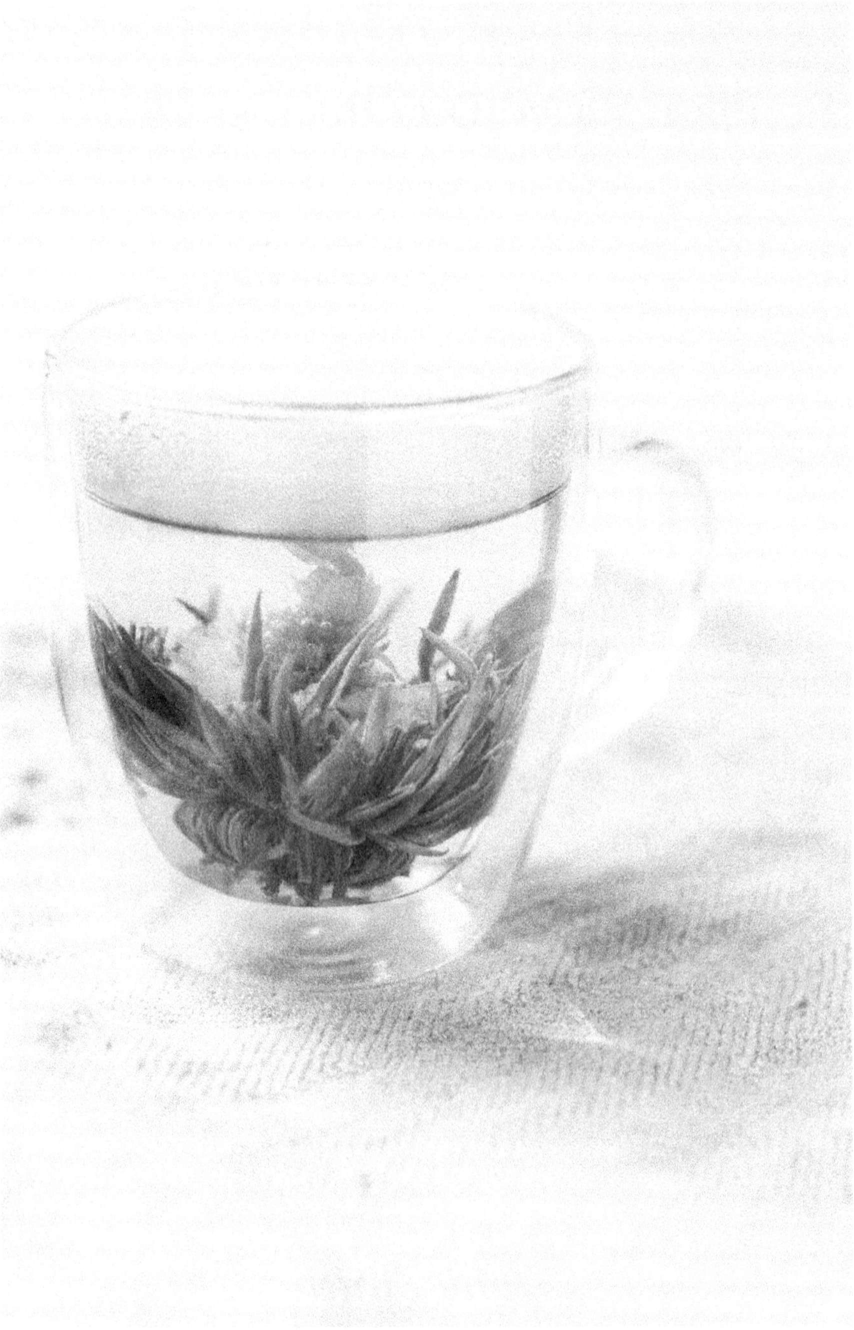

Breakfasts

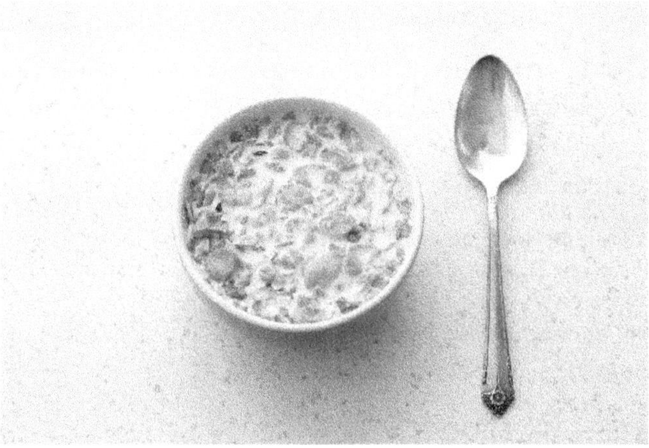

101 Onion & Mushroom Tart with a Nice Brown Rice Crust

Preparation 10 minutesCooking 55 minutes Serving: 1

Ingredients:

1 ½ pounds, mushrooms, button, portabella, 1 cup, short-grain brown rice

2 ¼ cups, water

½ teaspoon, ground black pepper2 teaspoons, herbal spice blend 1 sweet large onion 7 ounces, extra-firm tofu

1 cup, plain non-dairy milk 2 teaspoons, onion powder

2 teaspoons, low-sodium soy1 teaspoon, molasses

¼ teaspoon, ground turmeric ¼ cup, white wine

¼ cup, tapiocaDirections:

Cook the brown rice and put it aside for later use.

Slice the onions into thin strips and sauté them in water until they aresoft. Then, add the molasses, and cook them for a few minutes.

Next, sauté the mushrooms in water with the herbal spice blend. Once the mushrooms are cooked and they are soft, add the white wine or sherry. Cook everything for a few more minutes.

In a blender, combine milk, tofu, arrowroot, turmeric, and onionpowder till you have a smooth mixture

On a pie plate, create a layer of rice, spreading evenly to form a crust. The rice should be warm and not cold. It will be easy to work with warm rice. You can also use a pastry roller to get an even crust. With your fingers, gently press the sides.

Take half of the tofu mixture and the mushrooms and spoon them over the tart dish. Smooth the level with your spoon.

Now, top the layer with onions followed by the tofu mixture. You can smooth the surface again with your spoon.

Sprinkle some black pepper on top.

Bake the pie at 350o F for about 45 minutes. Toward the end, you can cover it loosely with tin foil. This will help the crust to remain moist.

Allow the pie crust to cool down, so that you can slice it. If you are in love with vegetarian dishes, there is no way that you will not love thispie.

Nutrition: Calories: 245.3, Fats 16.4 g, Proteins 6.8 g, Carbohydrates 18.3 g

102 Perfect Breakfast Shake

Preparation: 5 minutesCooking: 0 minutes Servings: 2
Ingredients:

3 tablespoons, raw cacao powder1 cup, almond milk
2 frozen bananas

3 tablespoons, natural peanut butterDirections:
Use a powerful blender to combine all the ingredients. Process everything until you have a smooth shake.
Enjoy a hearty shake to kickstart your day.

Nutrition: Calories: 330, Fats 15 g, Carbohydrates 41 g, Proteins 11g

103 Beet Gazpacho

Preparation time: 10 minutesCooking time: 2 minutes Servings: 4
Ingredients:

½ large bunch young beets with stems, roots and leaves 2 small cloves garlic, peeled,
Salt to taste

Pepper to taste

½ teaspoon liquid stevia 1 glass coconut milk kefir1 teaspoon chopped dill
½ tablespoon canola oil

1 small red onion, chopped

1 tablespoon apple cider vinegar 2 cups vegetable broth or water 1 tablespoon chopped chives
1 scallion, sliced Roasted baby potatoesDirections:
Cut the roots and stems of the beets into small pieces. Thinly slicethe beet greens.

Place a saucepan over medium heat. Add oil. When the oil isheated, add onion and garlic and cook until onion turns translucent.

Stir in the beets, roots and stem and cook for a minute.

Add broth, salt and water and cover with a lid. Simmer until tender.

Add stevia and vinegar and mix well. Taste and adjust the stevia and vinegar if required.

Turn off the heat. Blend with an immersion blender until smooth.

Place the saucepan back over it. When it begins to boil, add beet greens and cook for a minute. Turn off the heat.

Cool completely. Chill if desired. Add rest of the ingredients and stir.
Serve in bowls with roasted potatoes if desired.

Nutrition: Calories 101, Fats 5 g, Carbohydrates 14 g, Proteins 2 g

104 Healthy Breakfast Bowl

Preparation: 10 mCooking: 10 m Ingredients:
1 vegan yogurt 1/2 avocado (peeled and diced) 1 handful blueberries 1 tablespoon cacao nibs 1 handful of strawberries 1 tablespoon mulberries 1 tablespoon goji berries tablespoon desiccated coconut

2 Directions:
Put the avocado in a nice bowl. Top up with vegan yogurt.

Sprinkle the remaining ingredients and enjoy it.

Nutrition: carbohydrates: 55 g calories: 471 Fat: 25g sodium: 183 g protein: 11 g sugar: 32 g

105 Pumpkin Pancakes

Preparation time: 15 minutesCooking time: 15 minutes Servings: 4
Ingredients

1 cups unsweetened almond milk1 teaspoon apple cider vinegar 2½ cups whole-wheat flour
2 tablespoons baking powder

½ Teaspoon baking soda1 teaspoon sea salt
1 teaspoon pumpkin pie spice or ½ teaspoon ground cinnamon plus¼ teaspoon grated nutmeg plus ¼ teaspoon ground allspice½ Cup canned pumpkin purée1 cup water tablespoon coconut oilDirections
In a small bowl, combine the almond milk and apple cider vinegar.Set aside.

In a bowl, whisk together the flour, baking powder, baking soda, salt,and pumpkin pie spice. In bowl, combine the almond milk mixture, pumpkin purée, and water, whisking to mix well. Mix the wet Ingredients to the dry Ingredients and fold together until the dry- Ingredients are just moistened.

In a nonstick pan or griddle over medium-high heat, melt the coconutoil and swirl to coat. Pour the batter into the pan ¼ cup at a time and cook until the pancakes are browned, about 5 minutes per side. Serve immediately.

106 Green Breakfast Smoothie

Preparation: 10 minutesCooking: 0 minutes Servings: 2
Ingredients

½ Banana, sliced cups spinach or other greens, such as kale 1 cup sliced berries of your choosing, fresh or frozen 1 orange, peeled and cut into segments
1 cup unsweetened nondairy milk cup ice Directions
In a blender, combine all the Ingredients.

Starting with the blender on low speed, begin blending the smoothie, gradually increasing blender speed until smooth. Serve immediately.

107 Blueberry And Chia Smoothie

Preparation: 10 minutesCooking: 0 minutes Servings: 2

Ingredients

1 tablespoons chia seeds 2 cups unsweetened nondairy milk 2 cups blueberries, fresh or frozen 2 tablespoons pure maple syrup or agave2 tablespoons cocoa powder

Directions:

Soak the chia seeds in the almond milk for 5 minutes.

In a blender, combine the soaked chia seeds, almond milk, blueberries, maple syrup, and cocoa powder and blend until smooth. Serve immediately.

108 Berries with Mascarpone on Toasted Bread

Preparation Time: 10 minutesCooking Time: 0 minute Servings: 1
Ingredients:

1 slice whole-wheat bread

2 tablespoons mascarpone cheese1/8 cup raspberries
1/8 cup strawberries

1 teaspoon fresh mint leavesDirections:
Spread the cheese on the bread.

Top with the berries and chopped mint leaves.Store in food container and refrigerate.
Toast in the oven when ready to eat.

Nutrition: Calories: 326 fat: 27.3g Saturated fat: 14.2g Cholesterol: 70mg Sodium: 130mg Potassium: 115mg Carbohydrates: 15.1g Fiber: 4.1g Sugar: 3g Protein: 7.9g

109 Fruit Cup

Preparation Time: 15 minutes Cooking Time: 0 minute Servings: 4 Ingredients:

2 cups melon, sliced

2 cups strawberries, sliced 2 cups grapes, sliced in half 2 cups peaches, sliced

3 tablespoons freshly squeezed lime juice

½ teaspoon ground ginger1 tablespoon honey
3 teaspoons lime zest

¼ cup coconut flakes, toastedDirections:
Toss the fruits in lime juice, ginger and honey.Sprinkle the lime zest on top. Top with the coconut flakes.

Nutrition: Calories: 65 Total fat: 1.3g Saturated fat: 1.1g Sodium: 20mg Potassium: 247mg Carbohydrates: 13.9g Fiber: 1.6g Sugar: 10g Protein: 1g

110 Oatmeal with Black Beans & Cheddar

Preparation Time: 10 minutesCooking Time: 0 minute Servings: 2
Ingredients:

½ cup rolled oats

¼ cup Vegan yogurt

½ cup almond milk

2 tablespoons seasoned black beans

2 tablespoons Cheddar cheese, shredded 1 stalk scallion, minced 1 tablespoon cilantro, chopped

Directions:

Mix all the ingredients except the cilantro in a glass jar with lid.Refrigerate for up to 5 days.
Sprinkle the cilantro on top before serving.

Nutrition: Calories: 47 Total fat: 1.2g Saturated fat: 0.5g Sodium: 30mg Potassium: 151mg Carbohydrates: 11g Fiber: 1.9g Sugar: 9g Protein: 2g

111Strawberry Smoothie Bowl

Preparation time: 30 minutesCooking time: 0 minutes Servings: 02
Ingredients:

Smoothie bowl:

1½ cups frozen strawberries

½ cup coconut milkChia seeds Directions:
In a blender jug, puree all the ingredients for the smooth bowl. Pour the smoothie in the serving bowl.
Add strawberries, banana and chia seeds on top.Chill well then serve.
Nutrition: Calories 275 Total Fat 14.5 g Saturated Fat 12.5 g

Cholesterol 36 mg Sodium 13 mg Total Carbs 25 g Fiber 5 g Sugar 5

g Protein 2.5 g

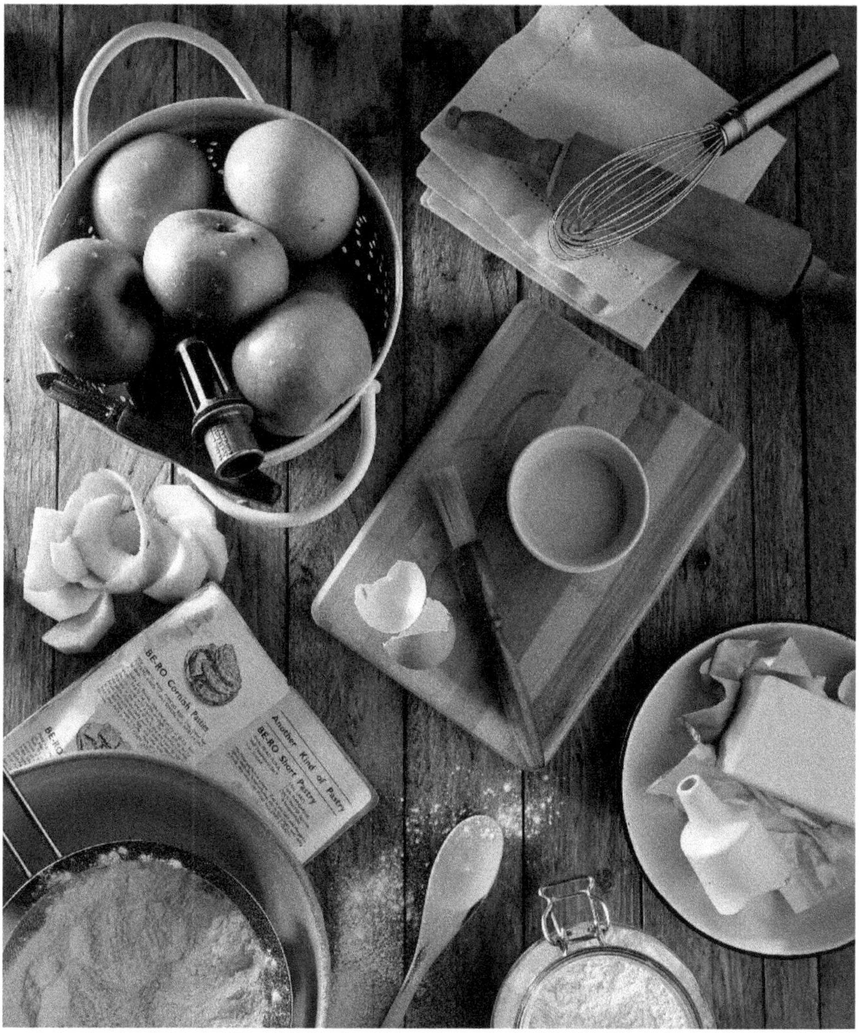
BE-RO Cornish Pasties
Another Kind of Pastry
BE-RO Short Pastry

Soups, Salads, and Sides

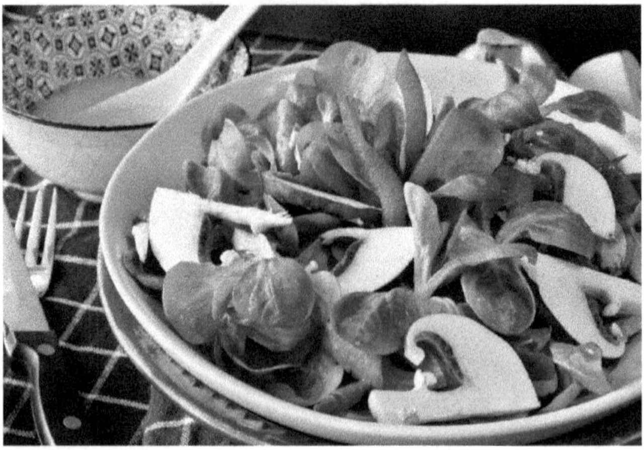

112 Creamy Squash Soup

Preparation time: 35 minutesCooking time: 22 minutes Servings: 8
Ingredients:

3 cups butternut squash, chopped

1 ½ cups unsweetened coconut milk1 tbsp coconut oil
1 tsp dried onion flakes1 tbsp curry powder
4 cups water

1 garlic clove

1 tsp kosher saltDirections:
Add squash, coconut oil, onion flakes, curry powder, water, garlic,and salt into a large saucepan. Bring to boil over high heat.

Turn heat to medium and simmer for 20 minutes.

Puree the soup using a blender until smooth. Return soup to the saucepan and stir in coconut milk and cook for 2 minutes.

Stir well and serve hot.

Nutrition: calories 146; fat 12.6 g; carbohydrates 9.4 g; sugar 2.8 g;

protein 1.7 g; cholesterol 0 mg

113 Cucumber Edamame Salad

Preparation time: 5 minutesCooking time: 8 minutes Servings: 2
Ingredients:

3 tbsp. Avocado oil

1 cup cucumber, sliced into thin rounds

½ cup fresh sugar snap peas, sliced or whole

½ cup fresh edamame

¼ cup radish, sliced

1 large avocado, peeled, pitted, sliced1 nori sheet, crumbled

2 tsp. Roasted sesame seeds1 tsp. Salt
Directions:

Bring a medium-sized pot filled halfway with water to a boil over medium-high heat.

Add the sugar snaps and cook them for about 2 minutes.

Take the pot off the heat, drain the excess water, transfer the sugar snaps to a medium-sized bowl and set aside for now.

Fill the pot with water again, add the teaspoon of salt and bring to aboil over medium-high heat.

Add the edamame to the pot and let them cook for about 6 minutes.

Take the pot off the heat, drain the excess water, transfer the soybeans to the bowl with sugar snaps and let them cool down for about 5 minutes.

Combine all ingredients, except the nori crumbs and roasted sesameseeds, in a medium-sized bowl.

Carefully stir, using a spoon, until all ingredients are evenly coated in oil. Top the salad with the nori crumbs and roasted sesame seeds.

Transfer the bowl to the fridge and allow the salad to cool for at least 30 minutes.

Serve chilled and enjoy!

Nutrition: Calories 409 Carbohydrates 7.1 g Fats 38.25 g Protein 7.6g

114 Best Broccoli Salad

Preparation time: 15 minutesChilling time: 1 hour Servings: 8
Ingredients:

8 cups diced broccoli

¼ cup sunflower seeds

3 tablespoons apple cider vinegar

½ cup dried cranberries1/3 cup cubed onion

1 cup mayonnaise

½ cup bacon bits

2 tablespoons sugar

½ teaspoon salt and ground black pepperDirections:
In a bowl, mix vinegar, salt, pepper, mayonnaise, and sugar. Mix it

well. In another bowl, mix all the remaining ingredients and pour the prepared mayonnaise dressing and mix it well. Before serving to refrigerate it for at least an hour.

Nutrition: Carbohydrates 17g, protein 6g, fats 26g, calories 317

Entrées

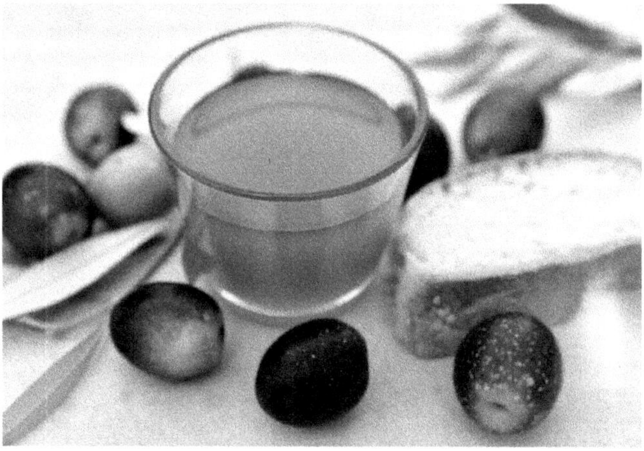

115 Crunchy Asparagus Spears

Preparation time: 25 minutesCooking time: 25 minutes Servings: 4
Ingredients:

1 bunch asparagus spears (about 12 spears)

¼ cup nutritional yeast

2 tablespoons hemp seeds1 teaspoon garlic powder
¼ teaspoon paprika (or more if you like paprika)

⅛ teaspoon ground pepper

¼ cup whole-wheat breadcrumbsJuice of ½ lemon
Directions:

Preheat the oven to 350 degrees, Fahrenheit. Line a ba

Wash the asparagus, snapping off the white part at the bottom. Save it for making vegetable stock.

Mix together the nutritional yeast, hemp seed, garlic powder, paprika, pepper and breadcrumbs.

Place asparagus spears on the baking sheets giving them a little room in between and sprinkle with the mixture in the bowl.

Bake for up to 25 minutes, until crispy.

Serve with lemon juice if desired.

116 Cucumber Bites with Chive and Sunflower Seeds

Preparation time: 5 minutesCooking time: 5 minutes Servings: 2
Ingredients:

1 cup raw sunflower seed ½ teaspoon salt

½ cup chopped fresh chives1 clove garlic, chopped

2 tablespoons red onion, minced

2 tablespoons lemon juice

½ cup water (might need more or less)4 large cucumbers

Directions:

Place the sunflower seeds and salt in the food processor and process to a fine powder. It will take only about 10 seconds.

Add the chives, garlic, onion, lemon juice and water and process until creamy, scraping down the sides frequently. The mixture should be very creamy; if not, add a little more water.

Cut the cucumbers into 1½-inch coin-like pieces.

Spread a spoonful of the sunflower mixture on top and set on a platter. Sprinkle more chopped chives on top and refrigerate until ready to serve.

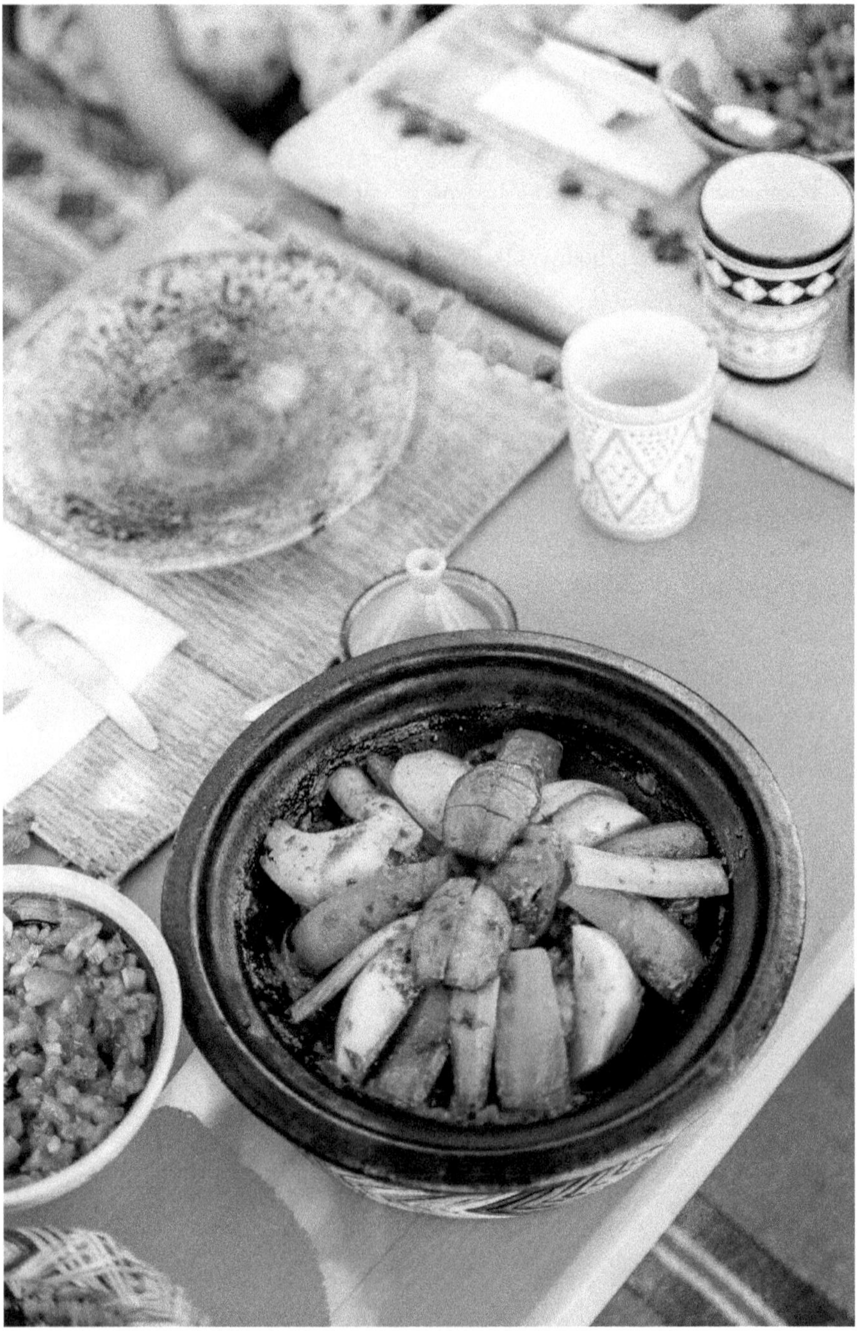

Smoothies and Beverages

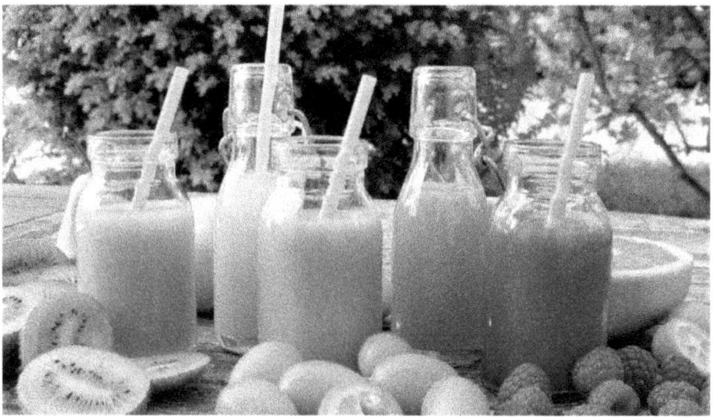

117 Tangy Spiced Cranberry Drink

Preparation time: 3 hours and 10 minutesCooking time: 3 hours
Servings: 14

Ingredients:

1 1/2 cups of coconut sugar12 whole cloves
2 fluid ounce of lemon juice

6 fluid ounce of orange juice

32 fluid ounce of cranberry juice8 cups of hot water
1/2 cup of Red Hot candies

Directions:

Pour the water into a 6-quarts slow cooker along with the cranberry juice, orange juice, and the lemon juice.

Stir the sugar properly.

Wrap the whole cloves in a cheese cloth, tie its corners with strings,and immerse it in the liquid present inside the slow cooker.

Add the red hot candies to the slow cooker and cover it with the lid.

Then plug in the slow cooker and let it cook on the low heat settingfor 3 hours or until it is heated thoroughly.

When done, discard the cheesecloth bag and serve.

Nutrition: Calories:89 Cal, Carbohydrates:27g, Protein:0g, Fats:0g, Fiber:1g.

118 Warm Pomegranate Punch

Preparation: 3 hours and 15 minutesCooking: 3 hours Servings: 10

Ingredients:

3 cinnamon sticks, each about 3 inches long12 whole cloves
1/2 cup of coconut sugar 1/3 cup of lemon juice

32 fluid ounce of pomegranate juice

32 fluid ounce of apple juice, unsweetened16 fluid ounce of brewed tea
Directions:

Using a 4-quart slow cooker, pour the lemon juice, pomegranate, juice apple juice, tea, and then sugar.

Wrap the whole cloves and cinnamon stick in a cheese cloth, tie its corners with a string, and immerse it in the liquid present in the slow cooker.

Then cover it with the lid, plug in the slow cooker and let it cook at the low heat setting for 3 hours or until it is heated thoroughly.

When done, discard the cheesecloth bag and serve it hot or cold.

Nutrition: Calories:253 Cal, Carbohydrates:58g, Protein:7g, Fats:2g, Fiber:3g.

119 Rich Truffle Hot Chocolate

Preparation time: 2 hours and 10 minutesCooking time: 2 hours
Servings: 4

Ingredients:

1/3 cup of cocoa powder, unsweetened1/3 cup of coconut sugar 1/8 teaspoon of salt

1/8 teaspoon of ground cinnamon

1 teaspoon of vanilla extract, unsweetened32 fluid ounce of coconut milk
Directions:

Using a 2 quarts slow cooker, add all the ingredients and stirproperly.

Cover it with the lid, then plug in the slow cooker and cook it for 2 hours on the high heat setting or until it is heated thoroughly.

When done, serve right away.

Nutrition: Calories:67 Cal, Carbohydrates:13g, Protein:2g, Fats:2g, Fiber:2.3g.

120 Vanilla Milkshake

Preparation: 5 min.Cooking: 5 min.Servings: 4
Ingredients:
2 c. ice cubes 2 t. vanilla extract

6 tbsp. powdered erythritol1 c. cream of dairy-free
½ c. coconut milkDirections:
In a high-speed blender, add all the ingredients and blend. Add ice cubes and blend until smooth.
Serve immediately and enjoy!

Nutrition: Calories: 125 | Carbohydrates: 6.8 g | Proteins: 1.2 g | Fats: 11.5 g

121 Raspberry Protein Shake

Preparation: 5 min. Cooking: 5 min.Serving: 1 Ingredients:
¼ avocado 1 c. raspberries, frozen1 scoop protein powder
½ c. almond milk

Ice cubes Directions:
In a high-speed blender add all the ingredients and blend until lumps of fruit disappear.

Add two to four ice cubes and blend to your desired consistency. Serve immediately and enjoy!
Nutrition: Calories: 756 | Carbohydrates: 80.1 g | Proteins: 27.6 g |

Fats: 40.7 g

122 Raspberry Almond Smoothie

Preparation: 5 min.Cooking: 5 min.Serving: 1

Ingredients:

10 Almonds, finely chopped3 tbsp. almond butter
1 c. almond milk 1 c. Raspberries, frozenDirections:
In a high-speed blender, add all the ingredients and blend until smooth.

Serve immediately and enjoy!

Nutrition: Calories: 449 | Carbohydrates: 26 g | Proteins: 14 g | Fats:35 g

123 Apple Raspberry Cobbler

Preparation Time: 50 minutesServings: 4

A safer type of fruit cobbler where a cut in sugar enhances the fruit. Ingredients

3 apples, peeled, cored, and chopped 2 tbsp pure date sugar cup fresh raspberries

1 tbsp unsalted plant butter

½ cup whole-wheat flour1 cup toasted rolled oats2 tbsp pure date sugar 1 tsp cinnamon powderDirections

Preheat the oven to 350 F and grease a baking dish with some plantbutter.

Add the apples, date sugar, and 3 tbsp of water to a medium pot. Cook over low heat until the date sugar melts and then, mix in the raspberries. Cook until the fruits soften, 10 minutes.

Pour and spread the fruit mixture into the baking dish and set aside. In a blender, add the plant butter, flour, oats, date sugar, and cinnamon powder. Pulse a few times until crumbly.

Spoon and spread the mixture on the fruit mix until evenly layered.Bake in the oven for 25 to 30 minutes or until golden brown on top.Remove the dessert, allow cooling for 2 minutes, and serve.

Nutritional info per serving

Calories 539 | Fats 12g| Carbs 105.7g | Protein 8.2g

Snacks and Desserts

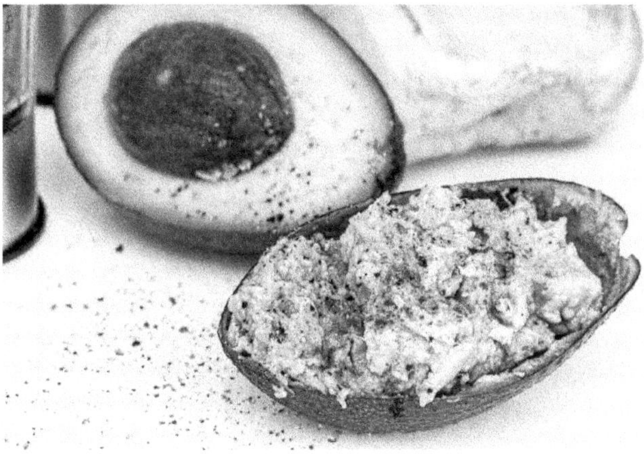

124 Simple Banana Fritters

Preparation time: 15 minsCooking time: 20 mins Servings: 8
Ingredients4 Bananas
3 Tbsps. Maple Syrup

¼ Tsp. Cinnamon Powder

¼ Tsp. Nutmeg

1 Cup Coconut FlourDirections
Preheat oven to 350° F.

Mash the bananas in a large mixing bowl along with maple syrup, cinnamon, nutmeg powder and coconut flour.

Mix all the ingredients well.

Take 2 tbsps. mixture and make small 1-inch-thick fritters from this mixture.

Place fritters in greased baking tray.

Bake fritters in preheated oven for about 10-15 minutes until golden from both sides.

Once done, take them out of the oven.Serve with coconut cream.
Enjoy!

Nutrition: Protein: 3% 3 kcal Fat: 28% 30 kcal Carbohydrates: 69% 75 kcal

125 Coconut And Blueberries Ice Cream

Preparation time: 5 minsCooking time: 0 mins Servings: 4
Ingredients

1/4 Cup Coconut Cream1 Tbsp. Maple Syrup
¼ Cup Coconut Flour

1 Cup Blueberries

¼ Cup Blueberries For ToppingDirections
Put ingredients into food processor and mix well on high speed.

Pour mixture in silicon molds and freeze in freezer for about 2-4 hours.

Once balls are set remove from freezer.Top with berries.
Serve cold and enjoy!

Nutrition: Protein: 3% 4 kcal Fat: 40% 60 kcal Carbohydrates: 57%

86 kcal

126 Peach Crockpot Pudding

Preparation time: 15 minsCooking time: 4 hours Servings: 6
Ingredients

2 Cups Sliced Peaches1/4 Cup Maple Syrup
1/2 Tsp. Cinnamon Powder

2 Cups Coconut MilkFor Serving
½ Cup Coconut Cream1 Oz. Coconut Flakes Directions
Lightly grease the crockpot and place peaches in the bottom. Add maple syrup, cinnamon powder and milk.
Cover and cook on high for 4 hours.

Once cooked remove from crockpot.For serving pour coconut cream.
Top with coconut flakes.Serve and enjoy!
Nutrition: Protein: 3% 11 kcal Fat: 61% 230 kcal Carbohydrates: 36%

133 kcal

127 Green Soy Beans Hummus

Preparation time: 15 minutesCooking time: 0 minutes Servings: 6
Ingredients

1 1/2 cups frozen green soybeans4 cups of water
coarse salt to taste

1/4 cup sesame paste 1/2 tsp grated lemon peel3 Tbsp fresh lemon juice
2 cloves of garlic crushed1/2 tsp ground cumin
1/4 tsp ground coriander

4 Tbsp extra virgin olive oil

1 Tbsp fresh parsley leaves chopped

Serving options: sliced cucumber, celery, olivesDirections:

1. In a saucepan, bring to boil 4 cups of water with 2 to 3 pinch of coarse salt.
2. Add in frozen soybeans, and cook for 5 minutes or until tender.
3. Rinse and drain soybeans into a colander.
4. Add soybeans and all remaining ingredients into a food processor.
5. Pulse until smooth and creamy.
6. Taste and adjust salt to taste.
7. Serve with sliced cucumber, celery, olives, bread...etc.

128 High Protein Avocado Guacamole

Preparation time: 15 minutesCooking time: 0 minutes Servings: 4
Ingredients

1/2 cup of onion, finely chopped

1 chili pepper (peeled and finely chopped) 1 cup tomato, finely chopped Cilantro leaves, fresh2 avocados

2 Tbsp linseed oil 1/2 cup ground walnuts1/2 lemon (or lime) Salt

Directions:

Chop the onion, chili pepper, cilantro, and tomato; place in a large bowl.

Slice avocado, open vertically, and remove the pit. Using the spoon take out the avocado flesh.

Mash the avocados with a fork and add into the bowl with onion mixture.

Add all remaining ingredients and stir well until ingredients combine well.

Taste and adjust salt and lemon/lime juice.

Keep refrigerated into covered glass bowl up to 5 days.

129 Homemade Energy Nut Bars

Preparation time: 15 minutesCooking time: 0 minutes Servings: 4
Ingredients

1/2 cup peanuts1 cup almonds
1/2 cup hazelnut, chopped

1 cup shredded coconut1 cup almond butter
2 tsp sesame seeds toasted

1/2 cup coconut oil, freshly melted2 Tbsp organic honey
1/4 tsp cinnamon

Directions

Add all nuts into a food processor and pulse for 1-2 minutes.

Add in shredded coconut, almond butter, sesame seeds, melted coconut oil, cinnamon, and honey; process only for one minute.

Cover a square plate/tray with parchment paper and apply the nut mixture.

Spread mixture vigorously with a spatula. Place in the freezer for 4 hours or overnight.
Remove from the freezer and cut into rectangular bars.

Ready! Enjoy!

130 Chocolate Energy Snack Bar

Preparation Time: 5 MinutesCooking Time: 0 Minutes

Servings: 4Ingredients:
Flax Seeds (1 T.)

Chia Seeds (1 T.) Agave Nectar (2 T.)Almonds (1 C.)
Dried Cranberries (1 C.)Dates (1 C.)
Directions:

When you need a snack that is easy to grab when you are on the go,this is the perfect recipe. You are going to start out by pulsing the almonds and dates in a food processor. Once they are chopped fine,add in the seeds, agave, and cranberries. At this point, pulse until everything is combined.

Next, you will want to add the batter into a lined pan and press everything down into the bottom.

Finally, pop the dish into the fridge for two hours, cut into squares, and your bars are ready!

Nutrition: Calories: 400 Proteins: 10g Carbs: 55g Fats: 20g

131 Zesty Orange Muffins

Preparation Time: 40 MinutesCooking Time: 20 Minutes Servings: 11
Ingredients:

Chopped Hazelnuts (3 T.)Orange Juice (1 C.)
Olive Oil (.50 C.)

Baking Powder (2 t.) Brown Sugar (.75 C.)Flour (2 C.)
Baking Soda (1 Pinch)Salt (to Taste)
Orange Zest (2 T.)

Directions:

Muffins are the perfect snack to grab and go when you need to leave the house quickly. Start off by prepping the oven to 350.

As this warms up, take out your mixing bowl and combine the hazelnuts, salt, baking soda, baking powder, sugar, and flour. Once these are mixed together well, add in the olive oil and orange juice.

With your mixture made, evenly pour into lined muffin tins and then pop it into the oven for 20 minutes.

By the end, the muffins should be cooked through and golden at the top. If they look done, remove from the oven, and your snack is ready to go.

Nutrition: Calories: 220 Proteins: 3g Carbs: 30g Fats: 10g

132 Chocolate Tahini Balls

Preparation Time: 10 MinutesCooking Time: 0 Minutes Servings: 8
Ingredients:

Sesame Seeds (2 T.)Tahini (2 T.)

Cacao Nibs (2 T.)

Unsweetened Cocoa Powder (2 T.) Old-fashioned Rolled Oats (.25 C.) Medjool Dates (4)
Rock Salt (1 Pinch)Directions:
For this quick snack, start off by placing all of the ingredients aboveinto a blender and blend until you get a dough-like texture.

Next, take the dough and mold it into 8 balls.

Place the balls in the fridge, allow to firm up for 20 minutes, and thenthey will be set.

Nutrition: Calories: 70 Proteins: 2g Carbs: 9g Fats: 4g

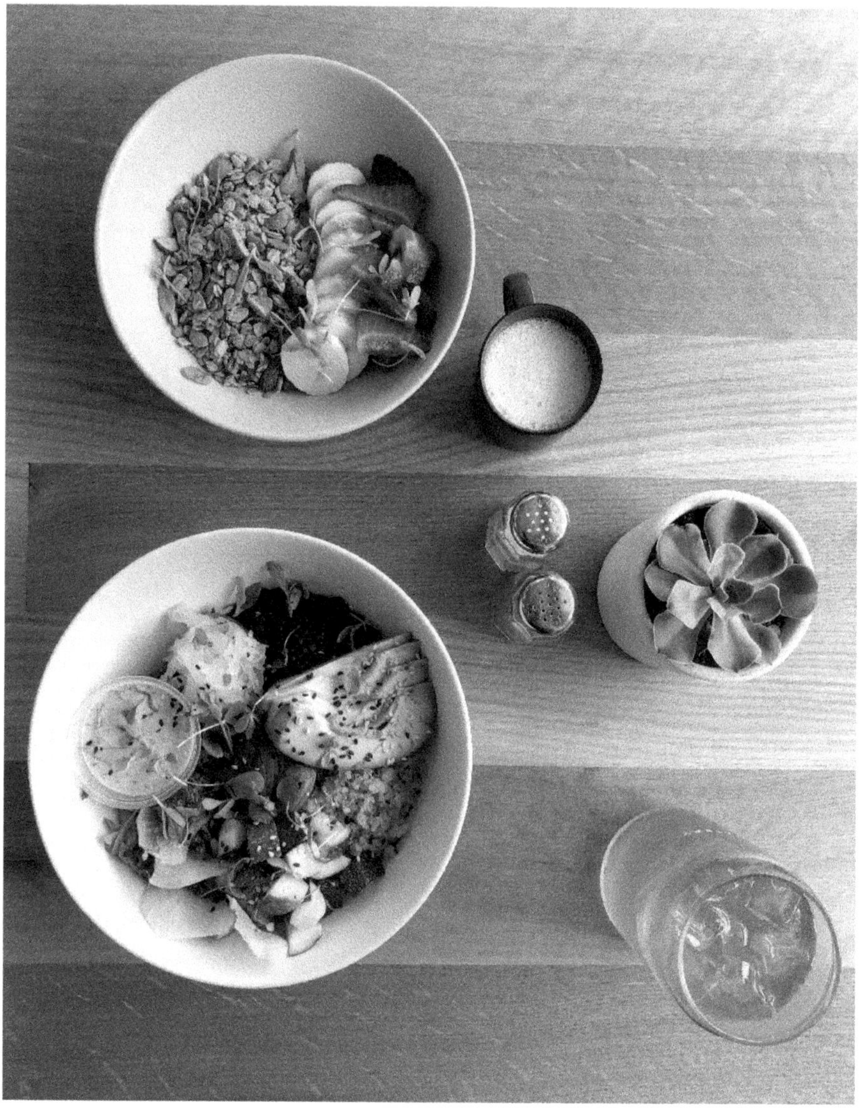

Dinner Recipes

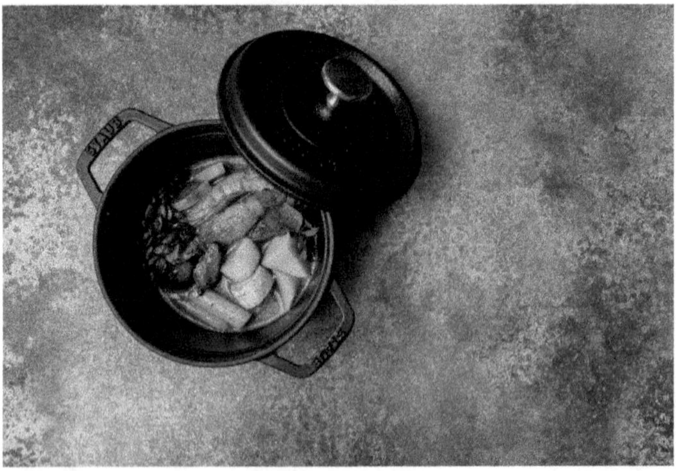

133 Piquillo Salsa Verde Steak

Preparation Time: 30 min.Cooking Time: 25 min.
Yields: 8 Servings

Ingredients:

4 – ½ inch thick slices of ciabatta18 oz. firm tofu, drained
5 tbsp. olive oil, extra virgin

Pinch of cayenne

½ t. cumin, ground

1 ½ tbsp. sherry vinegar1 shallot, diced
8 piquillo peppers (can be from a jar) – drained and cut to ½ inch strips

3 tbsp. of the following:

parsley, finely chopped capers, drained and choppedDirections:
Place the tofu on a plate to drain the excess liquid, and then sliceinto 8 rectangle pieces.

You can either prepare your grill or use a grill pan. If using a grill pan, preheat the grill pan.

Mix 3 tablespoons of olive oil, cayenne, cumin, vinegar, shallot, parsley, capers, and piquillo peppers in a medium bowl to make our salsa verde. Season to preference with salt and pepper.

Using a paper towel, dry the tofu slices.

Brush olive oil on each side, seasoning with salt and pepper lightly.

Place the bread on the grill and toast for about 2 minutes using medium-high heat.

Next, grill the tofu, cooking each side for about 3 minutes or until the tofu is heated through.

Place the toasted bread on the plate then the tofu on top of the bread.

Gently spoon out the salsa verde over the tofu and serve.

Nutrition: Calories: 427 | Carbohydrates: 67.5 g | Proteins: 14.2 g | Fats: 14.6 g

134 Sweet 'n spicy tofu

Preparation time 45 minutesCooking time: 10 minutes Servings: 8
Ingredients:

14 ounces extra firm tofu; press the excess liquid and chop into cubes.

3 tablespoons olive oil

2 2-3 cloves garlic, minced

4 tablespoons sriracha sauce or any other hot sauce 2 tablespoons soy sauce
1/4 cup sweet chili sauce

5-6 cups mixed vegetables of your choice (like carrots, cauliflower, broccoli, potato, etc.)

Salt to taste (optional)Direction:
Place a nonstick pan over medium-high heat. Add 1 tablespoon oil.

When oil is hot, add garlic and mixed vegetables and stir-fry until crisp and tender. Remove and keep aside.

Place the pan back on heat. Add 2 tablespoons oil. When oil is hot, add tofu and sauté until golden brown. Add the sautéed vegetables. Mix well and remove from heat.

Make a mixture of sauces by mixing together all the sauces in a small bowl.

Serve the stir fried vegetables and tofu with sauce.

Lunch Recipes

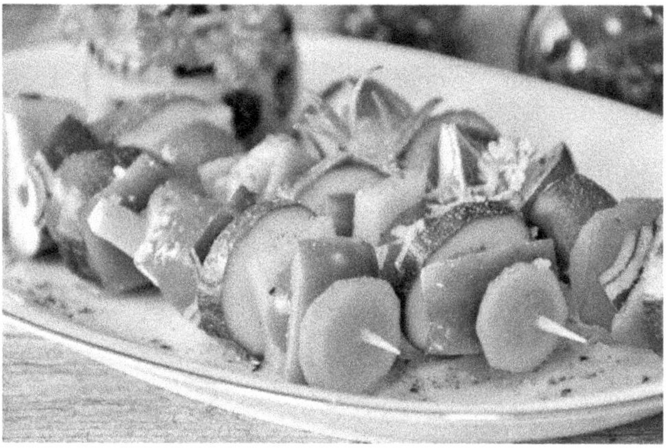

135 Green Pea Fritters

Preparation Time: 10 minutesCooking Time: 25 minutes Serving: 4
Ingredients:

For the Fritters:

1 ½ cups (140 grams) chickpea flour2 cups (250 grams) frozen peas
1 large white onion, peeled, diced

1 tablespoon minced garlic1/8 teaspoon salt
1 teaspoon baking soda

2 tablespoons mixed dried Italian herbs1 tablespoon olive oil
Water as needed

For the Yoghurt Sauce:

1/2 teaspoon dried rosemary 1/2 teaspoon dried parsley 1/2 teaspoon dried mint
1 lemon, juiced 1 cup soy yogurtDirections:
Switch on the oven, set it to 350° F and let it preheat.

Take a medium saucepan, place it over medium heat, add peas, cover them with water, bring it to a boil, cook for 2 to 3 minutes until tender, and when done, drain the peas and set aside until required.

Take a frying pan, place it over medium heat, add oil and when hot, add onion and garlic; cook for 5 minutes until softened.

Transfer onion-garlic mixture to a food processor, add peas and pulse for 1 minute until the thick paste comes together.

Tip the mixture in a bowl, add salt, baking soda, Italian herbs, and chickpea flour, stir until incorporated and shape the mixture into ten patties.

Brush the patties with oil, arrange them onto a baking sheet and bake for 15 to 18 minutes until golden brown and thoroughly cooked, turning halfway.

Meanwhile, prepare the yogurt sauce: take a medium bowl, add all the ingredients for it and whisk until combined.

Serve fritters with prepared yogurt sauce.

Nutrition: 94 Cal; 2 g Fat; 0 g Saturated Fat; 14 g Carbs; 3 g Fiber; 4 g Protein; 2 g Sugar

136 Broccoli Rabe

Preparation Time: 15 minutesCooking Time: 15 minutes Servings: 8
Ingredients:

2 oranges, sliced in half1 lb. broccoli rabe
2 tablespoons sesame oil, toasted

Salt and pepper to taste

1 tablespoon sesame seeds, toastedDirection
Pour the oil into a pan over medium heat.

Add the oranges and cook until caramelized.Transfer to a plate.
Put the broccoli in the pan and cook for 8 minutes.Squeeze the oranges to release juice in a bowl.
Stir in the oil, salt and pepper.

Coat the broccoli rabe with the mixture.Sprinkle seeds on top.
Nutrition: Calories: 59 Total fat: 4.4g Saturated fat: 0.6g Sodium:

164mg Potassium: 160mg Carbohydrates: 4.1g Fiber: 1.6g Sugar: 2g Protein: 2.2g

137 Whipped Potatoes

Preparation Time: 20 minutesCooking Time: 35 minutes Servings: 10
Ingredients:

4 cups water

3 lb. potatoes, sliced into cubes3 cloves garlic, crushed
6 tablespoons vegan butter2 bay leaves
10 sage leaves

½ cup Vegan yogurt

¼ cup low-fat milkSalt to taste Direction
Boil the potatoes in water for 30 minutes or until tender.Drain.
In a pan over medium heat, cook the garlic in butter for 1 minute.

Add the sage and cook for 5 more minutes.Discard the garlic.
Use a fork to mash the potatoes.

Whip using an electric mixer while gradually adding the butter, yogurt, and milk.

Season with salt.

Nutrition: Calories: 169 Total fat: 7.6g Saturated fat: 4.7g Cholesterol: 21mg Sodium: 251mg Potassium: 519mg Carbohydrates: 22.1g Fiber: 1.5g Sugar: 2g Protein: 4.2g

138 Chickpea Avocado Sandwich

You can make the chickpea and avocado filling ahead of time and store it in the cold-storage box for or in the icebox. While avocado does brown easily, the lime juice helps preserve the integrity of it.

Preparation time: 10 minutesCooking Time: 5 minutes Servings: 2
Ingredients: Chickpeas – 1 canAvocado – 1
Dill, dried – .25 teaspoon Onion powder – .25 teaspoon Sea salt – .5 teaspoon Celery, chopped – .25 cup
Green onion, chopped – .25 cupLime juice – 3 tablespoons Garlic powder – .5 teaspoon Dark pepper, ground – dash Tomato, sliced – 1
Lettuce – 4 leavesBread – 4 slices Directions:

Drain the canned chickpeas and rinse them under cool water. Place them in a bowl along with the herbs, spices, sea salt, avocado, and lime juice. Using a potato masher or fork, mash the avocado and chickpeas together until you have a thick filling. Try not to mash the chickpeas all the way, as they create texture.Stir the celery and green onion into the filling and prepare yoursandwiches.

Layout two slices of bread, top them with the chickpea filling, some lettuce, and sliced tomato. Top them off with the two remainingslices, slice the sandwiches in half, and serve. Nutrition: Calories 471

139 Pizza Bites

Preparation Time: 1 Hour Cooking Time: 30 MinutesServings: 4
Ingredients:

Olive Oil (1 t.)

Dried Oregano (1 t.) Lemon Juice (1 t.) Dried Basil (1 t.) Tomato Sauce (1 C.)Cauliflower (1 Head)Salt (to Taste)
Nutritional Yeast (to Taste)Garlic Cloves (2, Minced) Directions:
Begin by prepping the oven to 300 and line a pan with parchment paper. When this is set, take a mixing bowl and combine the olive oil,oregano, basil, salt, tomato sauce, and the basil together. In a second bowl, you will want to place your nutritional yeast.

When you are ready, gently dip the cauliflower pieces into the tomatosauce and then roll in the nutritional yeast. You will want to place these on the baking sheet and continue until all of the cauliflower is covered.

Once the cauliflower is set, place it into the oven for about an hour oruntil the edges are crispy. Once they are cooked to your liking, remove from the oven and enjoy with some extra sauce for dipping!

Nutrition: Calories: 110 Proteins: 5g Carbs: 17g Fats: 3g

140 Avocado, Spinach and Kale Soup

Preparation time: 10 minutesCooking time: 0 minutes Servings: 4
Ingredients:

2 avocados, pitted, peeled and cut in halves4 cups vegetable stock
2 tablespoons cilantro, chopped

Juice of 1 lime

1 teaspoon rosemary, dried

½ cup spinach leaves

½ cup kale, torn

Salt and black pepper to the tasteDirections:
In a blender, combine the avocados with the stock and the other ingredients, pulse well, divide into bowls and serve for lunch.

Nutrition: calories 300, fat 23, fiber 5, carbs 6, protein 7

141 Curry spinach soup

Preparation: 10 minutesCooking: 0 minutes Servings: 4

Ingredients:
1 cup almond milk

1 tablespoon green curry paste1 pound spinach leaves
1 tablespoon cilantro, chopped

Salt and black pepper to the taste4 cups veggie stock

2 tablespoon cilantro, choppedDirections:
In your blender, combine the almond milk with the curry paste and the other ingredients, pulse well, divide into bowls and serve for lunch. Nutrition: calories 240, fat 4, fiber 2, carbs 6, protein 2

142 Hot roasted peppers cream

Preparation: 10 minutes Cooking: 30 minutesServings: 4
Ingredients:

1 red chili pepper, minced4 garlic cloves, minced

2 pounds mixed bell peppers, roasted, peeled and chopped 4 scallions, chopped1 cup coconut cream
Salt and black pepper to the taste2 tablespoons olive oil
½ tablespoon basil, chopped4 cups vegetable stock
¼ cup chives, chopped

Directions:

Heat up a pot with the oil over medium heat, add the garlic and the chili pepper and sauté for 5 minutes.

Add the peppers and the other ingredients, toss, bring to a simmerand cook over medium heat for 25 minutes.

Blend the soup using an immersion blender, divide into bowls and serve.

Nutrition: calories 140, fat 2, fiber 2, carbs 5, protein 8

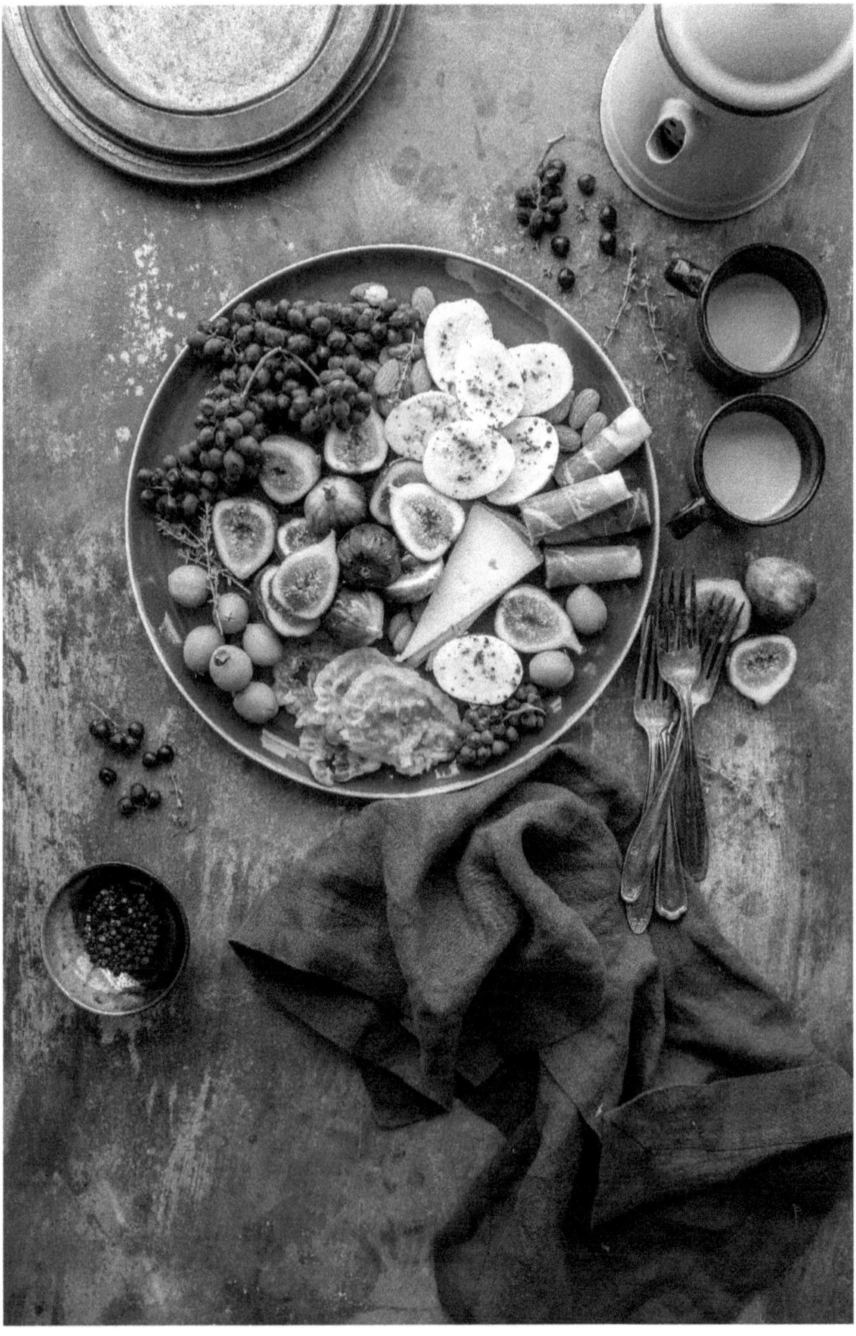

Recipes For Main Courses And Single Dishes

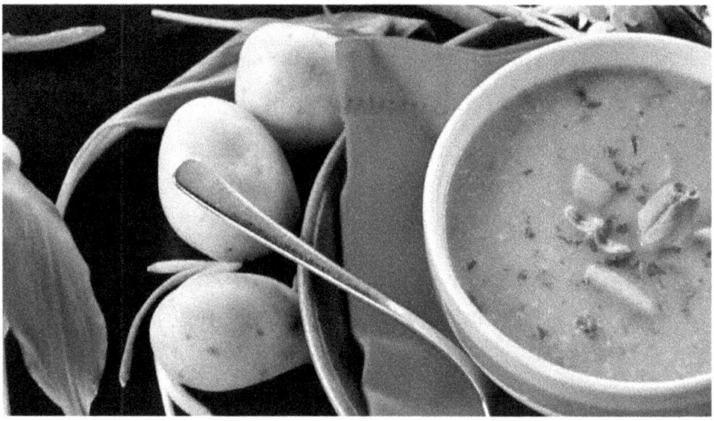

143 Smoked Tempeh with Broccoli Fritters

Preparation Time: 25 minutesCooking Time: 20 minutes Servings: 4
Ingredients:

For the flax egg:

4 tbsp flax seed powder + 12 tbsp waterFor the grilled tempeh:
3 tbsp olive oil

1 tbsp soy sauce

3 tbsp fresh lime juice1 tbsp grated ginger
Salt and cayenne pepper to taste10 oz. tempeh slices
For the broccoli fritters:

2 cups of rice broccoli8 oz. tofu cheese
3 tbsp plain flour

½ tsp onion powder1 tsp salt
¼ tsp freshly ground black pepper4¼ oz. vegan butter
For serving:

½ cup mixed salad greens1 cup vegan mayonnaise
½ lemon, juicedDirections:
For the smoked tempeh:

In a bowl, mix the flax seed powder with water and set aside to soak for 5 minutes.In another bowl, combine the olive oil, soy sauce, lime juice, grated ginger, salt, and cayenne pepper. Brush the tempeh slices with the mixture.

Heat a grill pan over medium heat and grill the tempeh on both sidesuntil nicely smoked and golden brown, 8 minutes. Transfer to a plate and set aside in a warmer for serving.

In a medium bowl, combine the broccoli rice, tofu cheese, flour, onion, salt, and black pepper. Mix in the flax egg until well combine and form 1-inch thick patties out of the mixture.

Melt the vegan butter in a medium skillet over medium heat and fry the patties on both sides until golden brown, 8 minutes. Remove the fritters onto a plate and set aside.

In a small bowl, mix the vegan mayonnaise with the lemon juice.

Divide the smoked tempeh and broccoli fritters onto serving plates, add the salad greens, and serve with the vegan mayonnaise sauce.

144 Cheesy Potato Casserole

Preparation Time: 30 minutesCooking Time: 20 minutes Servings: 4
Ingredients:

2 oz. vegan butter

½ cup celery stalks, finely chopped1 white onion, finely chopped

1 green bell pepper, seeded and finely choppedSalt and black pepper to taste

2 cups peeled and chopped potatoes1 cup vegan mayonnaise
4 oz. freshly shredded vegan Parmesan cheese1 tsp red chili flakes
Directions:

Preheat the oven to 400 F and grease a baking dish with cooking spray.

Season the celery, onion, and bell pepper with salt and blackpepper.

In a bowl, mix the potatoes, vegan mayonnaise, Parmesan cheese,and red chili flakes.

Pour the mixture into the baking dish, add the season vegetables,and mix well.

Bake in the oven until golden brown, about 20 minutes. Remove the baked potato and serve warm with baby spinach.

145 Curry Mushroom Pie

Preparation Time: 65 minutesCooking Time: 1 hour Servings: 4
Ingredients:

For the piecrust:

1 tbsp flax seed powder + 3 tbsp water

¾ cup plain flour 4 tbsp. chia seeds
4 tbsp almond flour

1 tbsp nutritional yeast1 tsp baking powder
1 pinch salt

3 tbsp olive oil4 tbsp water For the filling:
1 cup chopped baby Bella mushrooms1 cup vegan mayonnaise

4 tbsp + 9 tbsp water

½ red bell pepper, finely chopped1 tsp curry powder
½ tsp paprika powder ½ tsp garlic powder

¼ tsp black pepper ½ cup coconut cream

1¼ cups shredded vegan Parmesan cheeseDirections:
In two separate bowls, mix the different portions of flaxseed powder with the respective quantity of water. Allow soaking for 5 minutes.

For the piecrust:

Preheat the oven to 350 F.

When the flax egg is ready, pour the smaller quantity into a food processor and pour in all the ingredients for the piecrust. Blend until soft, smooth dough forms.

Line an 8-inch springform pan with parchment paper and grease with cooking spray.

Spread the dough in the bottom of the pan and bake for 15 minutes. For the filling:
In a bowl, add the remaining flax egg and all the filling's ingredients.Combine well and pour the mixture on the piecrust. Bake further for40 minutes or until the pie is golden brown.

Remove from the oven and allow cooling for 1 minute.Slice and serve the pie warm.

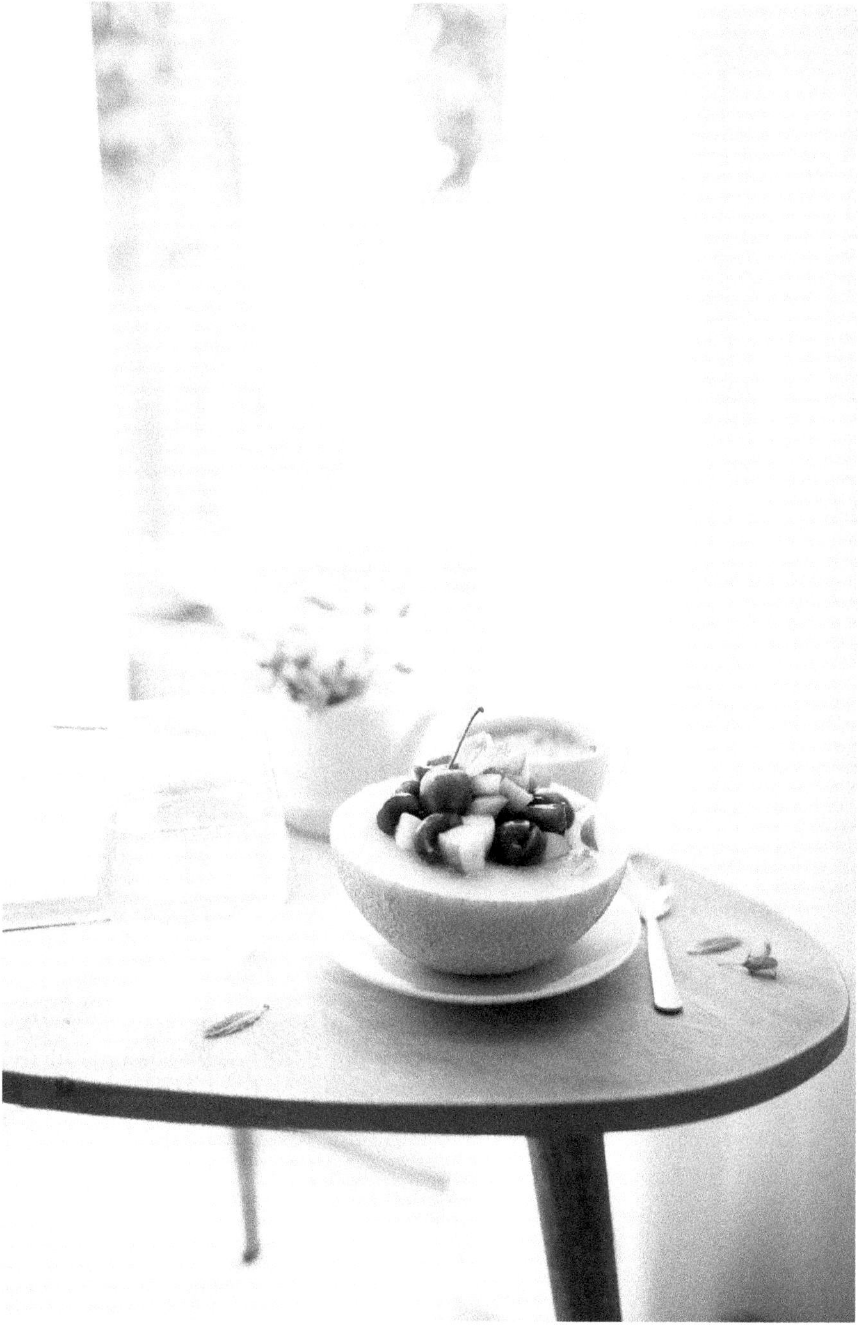

Nutrient-Packed Protein Salads

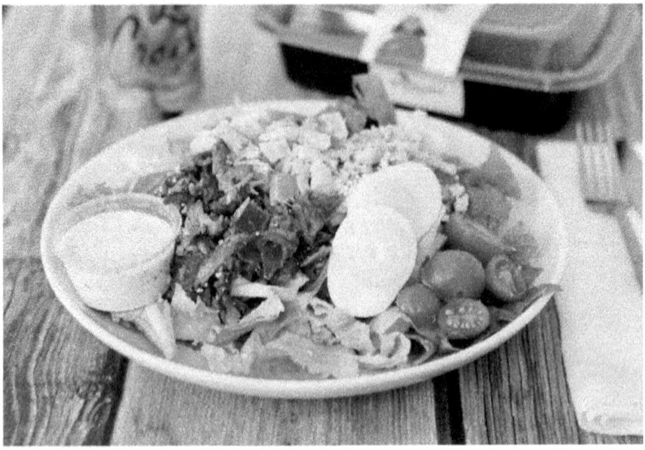

146 Arugula Lentil Salad

Preparation time: 5 mins.Cooking time: 5 mins.

Ingredient: ¾ cups cashews (¾ cups = 100 g)1 onion

3 tbsp olive oil

1 chilli / jalapeño

5-6 sun-dried tomatoes in oil3 slices bread (whole wheat)

1 cup brown lentils, cooked (1 cup = 1 / 15oz / 400 g)

1 handful arugula/rocket (1 handful = 100 g)1-2 tbsp balsamic vinegar salt and pepper to taste.

Directions:

Roast the cashews on a low heat for about three minutes in a pan to maximize aroma. Then throw them into the salad bowl. Dice up and fry the onion in one third of the olive oil for about 3 minutes on a low heat. Meanwhile chop the chilli/jalapeño and dried tomatoes. Add them to the pan and fry for another 1-2 minutes. Cut the bread into big croutons. Move the onion mix into a big bowl. Now add the restof the oil to the pan and fry the chopped-up bread until crunchy. Season with salt and pepper. Wash the arugula and add it to the bowl. Put the lentils in too, and mix them all around. Season withsalt, pepper and balsamic vinegar. Serve with the croutons. Super tasty!

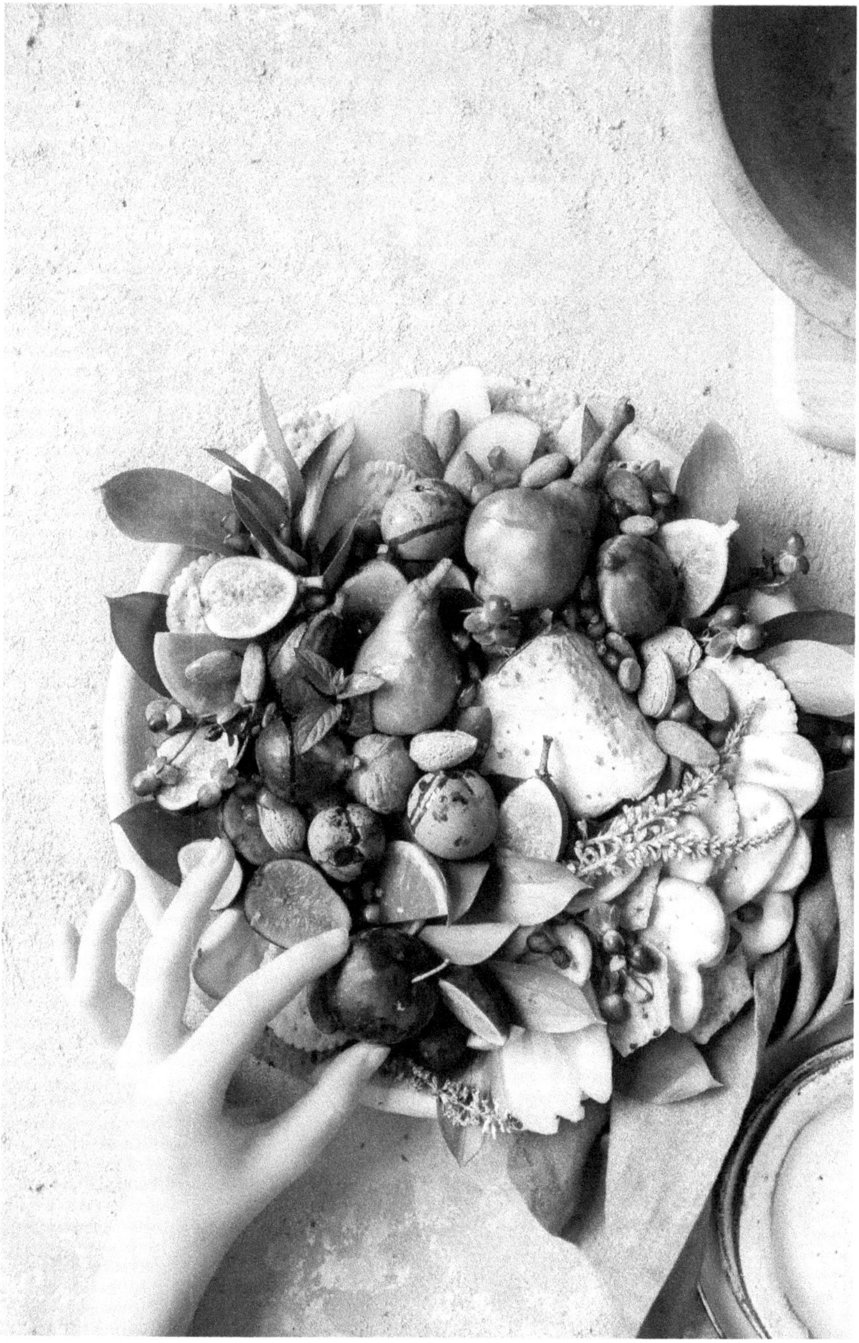

Flavour Boosters (Fish Glazes, Meat Rubs & Fish Rubs)

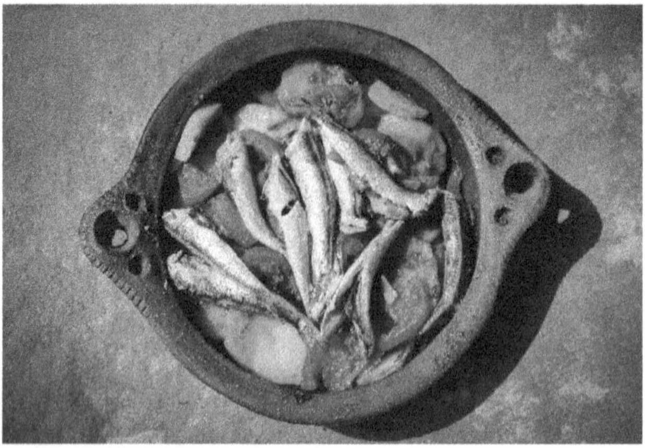

147 Tunisian Mixed Spiced Rub

This incredible rub recipe hailed from the Tunisian cooking secrets; the rub is the essential seasoning base for variety of Tunisian dishes.

This lovely spice blend created by caraway seeds, coriander, and hotpepper works like a charm on your favorite pork tenderloin, chicken as well as salmon.

Preparation Time: 5 min.Cooking Time: 5 min.
Servings: 5-½ tsp.Ingredients:

Coriander seeds - 2 tsp. Caraway seeds - 2 tsp. Crushed red pepper - 3/4 tsp.Garlic powder - 3/4 tsp.
Kosher salt - 1/2 tsp.Directions:
Mix in the coriander seeds, red pepper and caraway seeds in your spice blender, grinder or processor to make this rub. Start processing or blending the mixed spices on "pulse" mode mixture to ground.

Put the mixed spice mixture into a bowl; mix in the salt and garlic powder. Mix again well.

Now, take your choice of meat cut and place it on a firm surface. Brush or rub the freshly made rub on it; pat gently for the rub to stick onto the surface. Turn the meat cut and repeat to spice up its other side. Repeat with other meat cuts.

The freshly rubbed meat is ready to be grilled or cooked!

148 All Purpose Dill Seed Rub

Boost your steak with vibrant, spiced flavors of this all-purpose dill seed rub. It also beautifully seasons chicken and pork meat cuts. Apply this unique rub minutes before grilling or cooking; you can alsostore it at room temperature for 12-14 days without sacrificing on its quality.

Preparation Time: 5 min.Cooking Time: 5 min.
Servings: 6-7 tsp.

Ingredients:

Paprika - 2 tsp.

Ground coriander - 2 tsp.Dill seed – 1 tsp.
Dry mustard - ½ tsp. Garlic, minced – 1 clove
Black pepper and salt as requiredCayenne pepper - ¼ tsp.
Directions:

Mix in all the rub ingredients in your mixing bowl to make the dill seed rub. Gently mix all ingredients using spatula or spoon to forman aromatic rub mixture.

Now, take your choice of meat cut and place it on a firm surface. Brush the freshly made rub on it; pat gently for the rub to stick onto the surface. Turn the meat cut and repeat to spice up its other side. Repeat with other meat cuts.

Let your meat cuts adequately season for more rich flavors for a few hours in your refrigerator. Take them out, as they are ready to be cooked or grilled!

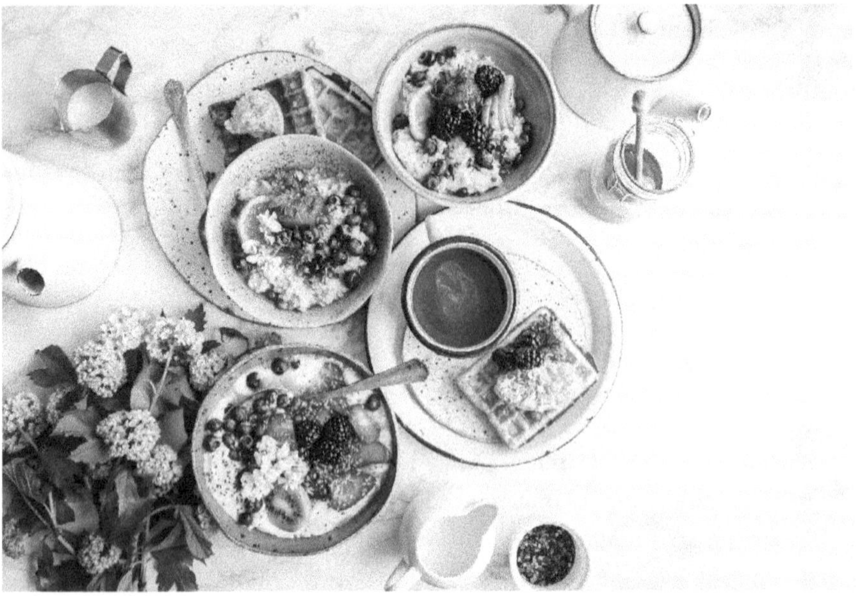

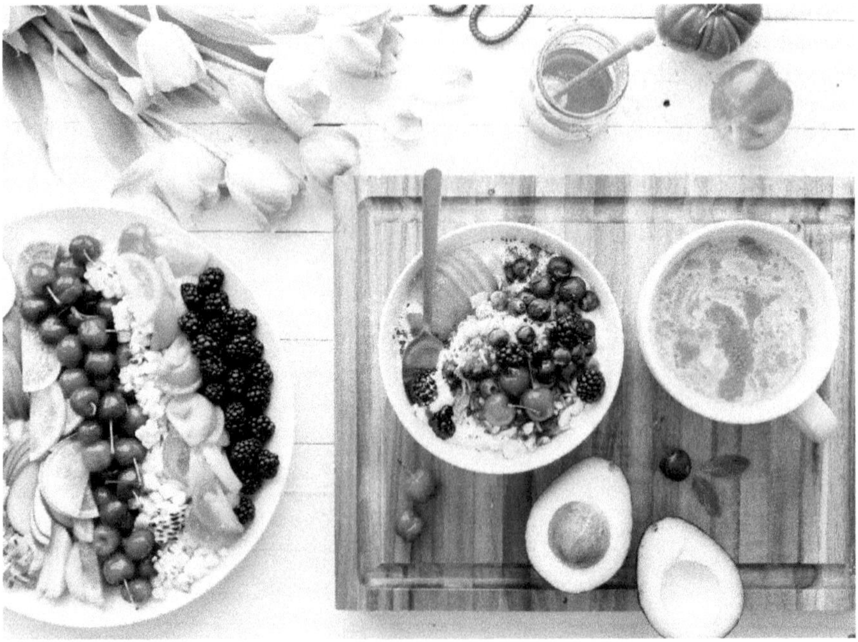

Sauce Recipes

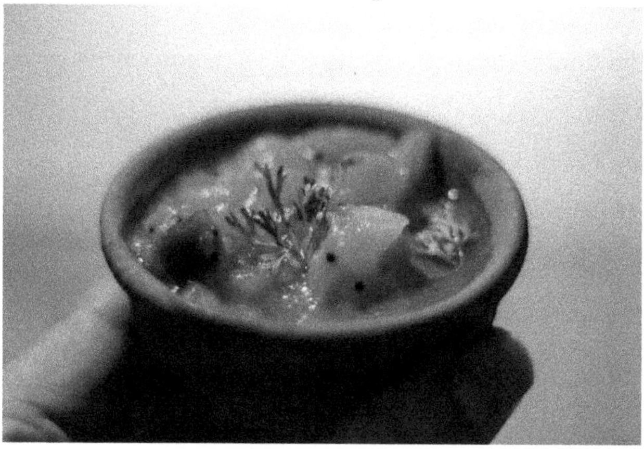

149 Vegan Ranch Dressing (Dipping Sauce)

Preparation time: 5 minutesCooking time: 5 minutes Servings: 8
Ingredients:

1 tablespoons lemon juice14 oz. silken tofu
1 tablespoon yellow mustard

1 tablespoon apple cider vinegar1 teaspoon onion granules
1 tablespoon agave

1 teaspoon garlic granules

2 tablespoons parsley, minced2 tablespoons dill, minced
1/2 teaspoon Himalayan salt

Directions:

Add all ingredients except parsley and dill to a blender and blend until smooth at high speed.

Add dill and parsley and blend until mixed.Serve chilled.

150 Vegan Smokey Maple BBQ Sauce

Preparation time: 5 minutesCooking time: 5 minutes Servings: 8
Ingredients:

1 tablespoon maple syrup1/2 cup ketchup
1 teaspoon garlic powder1 teaspoon liquid smoke Directions:
Add all ingredients to a bowl. Mix them until well combined. Serve and enjoy.

The Complete Plant Based Diet Cookbook

Healthy and Delicious Recipes to Lose Weight Feel Great on a Budget

Frank Smith

Breakfasts

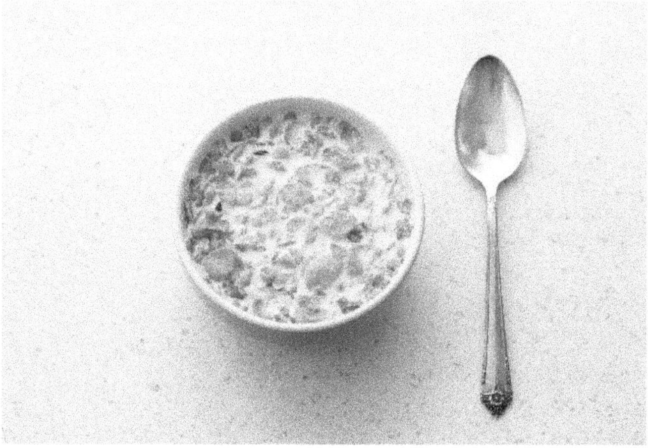

151 Oatmeal Fruit Shake

Preparation Time: 10 minutesCooking time: 0 minutes Servings: 2
Ingredients:

1 cup oatmeal, already prepared, cooled1 apple, cored, roughly chopped
1 banana, halved

3 cup baby spinach 2 cups coconut water2 cups ice, cubed
½ tsp ground cinnamon 1 tsp pure vanilla extractDirections:
Add all ingredients to a blender.

Blend from low to high for several minutes until smooth.

Nutrition: Calories 270 Carbohydrates 58 g Fats 1.5 g Protein 5 g

152 Amaranth Banana Breakfast Porridge

Preparation Time: 10 minutesCooking time: 25 minutes Servings: 8
Ingredients:

4 cup amaranth

2 cinnamon sticks

4 bananas, diced

2 Tbsp chopped pecans4 cups water
Directions:

Combine the amaranth, water, and cinnamon sticks, and banana in apot. Cover and let simmer around 25 minutes.

Remove from heat and discard the cinnamon. Places into bowls, andtop with pecans.

Nutrition: Calories 330 Carbohydrates 62 g Fats 6 g Protein 10 g

153 Green Ginger Smoothie

Preparation time: 5 minutesCooking time: 5 minutes Servings: 2
Ingredients:

1 banana

½ apple sliced

3 orange sliced and peeled1 lemon juice
4 big spinach

1 tbsp. fresh ginger

½ cup almond milk

For the dressing: chia seeds, apple, raspberriesDirections:
Take a blender. Peel off and slice all fruits. Add banana, apple, orange, lime juice, ginger and spinach and blend them well until theyturn smooth. Now add almond milk and pulse again for a few seconds. Pour the smoothie into glasses and serve. You can add chia seeds, apple or raspberries for a smoothie bowl. Store it up to 8-10 hours in the refrigerator.

Nutrition: Calories 330 Carbohydrates 62 g Fats 6 g Protein 10 g

154 Chocolate Strawberry Almond Protein Smoothie

Preparation time: 10 mCooking time: 10 m Ingredients:
1 cup of organic strawberries

1 1/2 cup homemade almond milk 1 scoop chocolate protein powder 1 tablespoon organic coconut oil 1/4 cup organic raw almonds

3 tablespoon organic hemp seeds 1 tablespoon organic maca powderFor Garnish:
organic cacao nibs organic hemp seedsDirections:
Put all the ingredients inside a blender and beat until they are well combined.

Optional: Garnish with organic hemp seeds or organic cocoa beans.Enjoy it!
Nutrition: carbohydrates: 39 g calories: 720 Fat: 45 g sodium: 732g

protein: 44 g sugar: 12g

155 Apple and Cinnamon Oatmeal

Preparation time: 10 minutesCooking time:10 minutes Servings: 2
Ingredients

1¼ cups apple cider

1 apple, peeled, cored, and chopped

⅔ Cup rolled oats

1 teaspoon ground cinnamon

1 tablespoon pure maple syrup or agave (optional)Directions
In a medium saucepan, bring the apple cider to a boil over medium-high heat. Stir in the apple, oats, and cinnamon.

Bring the cereal to a boil and turn down heat to low. Simmer until the oatmeal thickens, 3 to 4 minutes. Spoon into two bowls and sweeten with maple syrup, if using. Serve hot.

156 13 bis. Mango Key Lime Pie Smoothie

Preparation time: 5 minutesCooking time: 0 minutes Servings: 1
Ingredients

¼ Avocado 1 cup baby spinach

½ Cup frozen mango chunks

1 cup unsweetened soy or almond milkJuice of 1 lime (preferably a key lime). 1 tablespoon maple syrup
Directions

Combine all the Ingredients in a blender and blend until smooth. Enjoy immediately.

157 Spiced Orange Breakfast Couscous

Preparation time: 10 minutesCooking time: 10 minutes Servings: 4
Ingredients

3 cups orange juice1½ cups couscous
1 teaspoon ground cinnamon

¼ Teaspoon ground cloves

½ Cup dried fruit, such as raisins or apricots

½ Cup chopped almonds or other nuts or seedsDirections
In a small saucepan, bring the orange juice to a boil. Add the couscous, cinnamon, and cloves and remove from heat. Cover the pan with a lid and allow to sit until the couscous softens, about 5 minutes.

Fluff the couscous with a fork and stir in the dried fruit and nuts. Serve immediately.

158 Fig & Cheese Oatmeal

Preparation Time: 10 minutesCooking Time: 0 minute Servings: 1
Ingredients:

½ cup water

½ cup rolled oatsPinch salt
2 tablespoons dried figs, sliced

2 tablespoons ricotta cheese

2 teaspoons agave syrup

3 tablespoon almonds, toasted and slicedDirections:
Put the water, oats and salt in a glass jar with lid.Shake to blend well.
Refrigerate for up to 5 days.

Top with the remaining ingredients when ready to serve.

Nutrition: Calories: 294 Total fat: 8.5g Saturated fat: 2.3g Cholesterol: 10mg Sodium: 182mg Potassium: 362mg Carbohydrates: 47.5g Fiber: 6.6g Sugar: 16g Protein: 10.4g

159 Pumpkin Oats

Preparation: 10 minutesCooking: 0 minute Servings: 1
Ingredients:

½ cup rolle oats ½ cup almond milk ¼ cup ricotta cheese

4 tablespoons pumpkin puree1 tablespoon maple syrup
¼ teaspoon vanilla 1/8 teaspoon ground nutmegDirections:
Combine all the ingredients in a glass jar with lid.

Refrigerate for up to 5 days. Nutrition: Calories: 344 Total fat: 10g Saturated fat: 3.8g Cholesterol: 19mg Sodium: 179mg Potassium: 364mg Carbohydrates: 51.7g Fiber: 5.7g Sugar: 16g Protein: 13.3g

160 Apple Chia Pudding

Preparation time: 10 minutesCooking time: 5 minutes Servings: 04
Ingredients:

Chia Pudding:

4 tablespoons chia seeds1 cup almond milk
½ teaspoon cinnamonApple Pie Filling:

3 large apple, peeled, cored and chopped

¼ cup water

4 teaspoons maple syrupPinch cinnamon
2 tablespoons golden raisinsDirections:
In a sealable container, add cinnamon, chia seeds and almond milk, mix well.

Seal the container and refrigerate overnight.

In a medium pot, combine all apple pie filling ingredients and cook for 5 minutes.

Serve the chia pudding with apple filling on top.Enjoy.
Nutrition: Calories387TotalFat5.8gSaturatedFat4.2 g

Cholesterol 41 mg Sodium 154 mg Total Carbs 24.1 g Fiber 2.9 g

Sugar 3.1 g Protein 6.6 g

Soups, Salads, and Sides

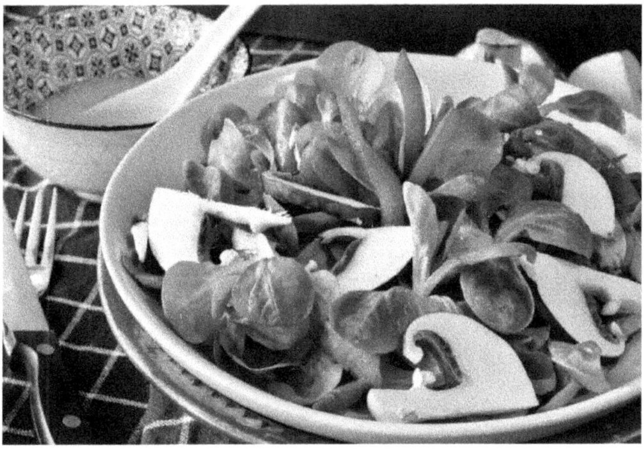

161 Garden PatchSandwichesonMultigrain Bread

Preparation time: 15 minutes Cooking time: 0 minutes Servings: 4 sandwiches Ingredients:

1pound extra-firm tofu, drained and patted dry1 medium red bell pepper, finely chopped

1 celery rib, finely chopped

5 green onions, minced

¼ cup shelled sunflower seeds

½ cup vegan mayonnaise, homemade or store-bought

½ teaspoon salt

½ teaspoon celery salt

¼ teaspoon freshly ground black pepper8 slices whole grain bread

6 (¼-inch) slices ripe tomato

4 lettuce leavesDirections:

Crumble the tofu and place it in a large bowl. Add the bell pepper, celery, green onions, and sunflower seeds. Stir in the mayonnaise, salt, celery salt, and pepper and mix until well combined.

Toast the bread, if desired. Spread the mixture evenly onto 4 slices of the bread. Top each with a tomato slice, lettuce leaf, and the remaining bread. Cut the sandwiches diagonally in half and serve.

162 Garden Salad Wraps

Preparation time: 15 minutesCooking time: 10 minutes Servings: 4 wraps
Ingredients:
6 tablespoons olive oil

2-pound extra-firm tofu, drained, patted dry, and cut into ½-inch strips

1 tablespoon soy sauce

¼ cup apple cider vinegar

1 teaspoon yellow or spicy brown mustard

½ teaspoon salt

¼ teaspoon freshly ground black pepper3 cups shredded romaine lettuce
3 ripe roma tomatoes, finely chopped

1 large carrot, shredded

1 medium english cucumber, peeled and chopped

⅓ cup minced red onion

¼ cup sliced pitted green olives

4 (10-inch) whole-grain flour tortillas or lavash flatbreadDirections:
In a large skillet, heat 2 tablespoons of the oil over medium heat. Add the tofu and cook until golden brown, about 10 minutes. Sprinkle with soy sauce and set aside to cool.

In a small bowl, combine the vinegar, mustard, salt, and pepper with the remaining 4 tablespoons oil, stirring to blend well. Set aside.

In a large bowl, combine the lettuce, tomatoes, carrot, cucumber, onion, and olives. Pour on the dressing and toss to coat.

To assemble wraps, place 1 tortilla on a work surface and spread with about one-quarter of the salad. Place a few strips of tofu on the tortilla and roll up tightly. Slice in half

163 Marinated Mushroom Wraps

Preparation time: 15 minutes Cooking time: 0 minutes Servings: 2 wraps
Ingredients:
3 tablespoons soy sauce

3 tablespoons fresh lemon juice

11/2 tablespoons toasted sesame oil

2 portobello mushroom caps, cut into 1/4-inch strips 1 ripe hass avocado, pitted and peeled
2 cups fresh baby spinach leaves

1 medium red bell pepper, cut into 1/4-inch strips1 ripe tomato, chopped
Salt and freshly ground black pepper

Directions:

In a medium bowl, combine the soy sauce, 2 tablespoons of the lemon juice, and the oil. Add the portobello strips, toss to combine, and marinate for 1 hour or overnight. Drain the mushrooms and set aside.

Mash the avocado with the remaining 1 tablespoon of lemon juice.

To assemble wraps, place 1 tortilla on a work surface and spread with some of the mashed avocado. Top with a layer of baby spinach leaves. In the lower third of each tortilla, arrange strips of the soaked mushrooms and some of the bell pepper strips. Sprinkle with the

tomato and salt and black pepper to taste. Roll up tightly and cut inhalf diagonally. Repeat with the remaining ingredients and serve.

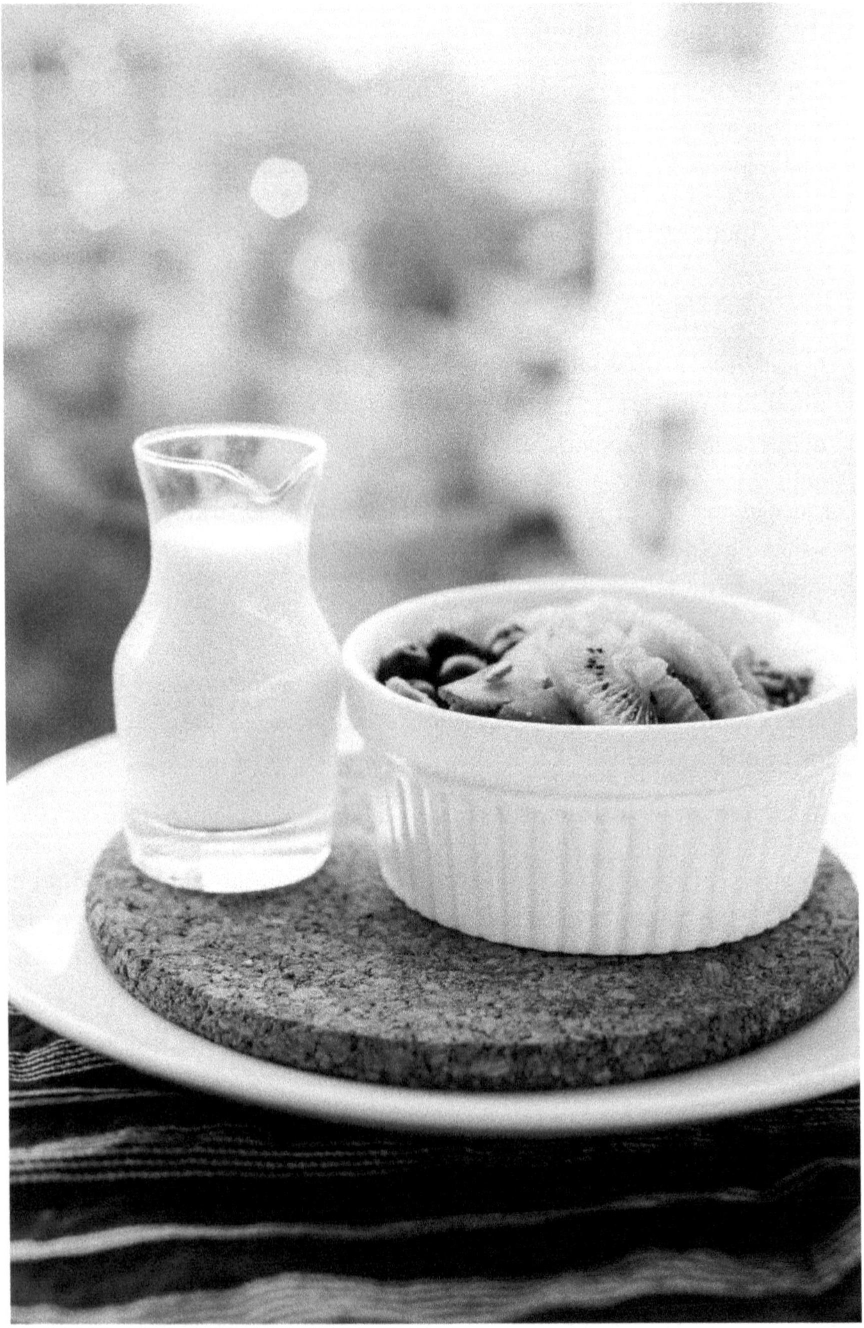

Entrées

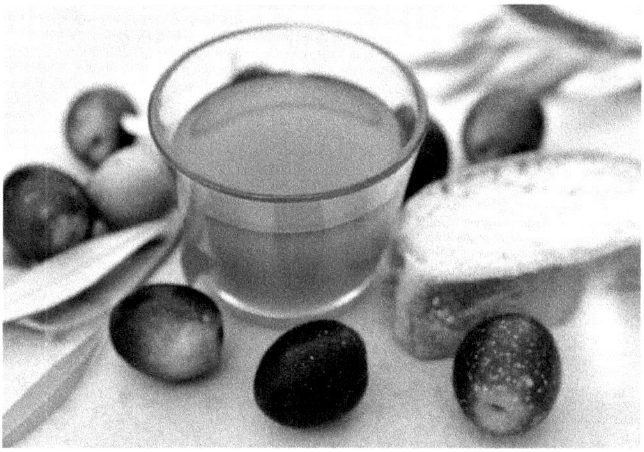

164 Homemade Trail Mix

Preparation time: 20 minutesCooking time: 20 minutes Servings: 2
Ingredients:

½ cup uncooked old-fashioned oatmeal

½ cup chopped dates

2 cups whole grain cereal

¼ cup raisins

¼ cup almonds

¼ cup walnutsDirections:
Mix all the ingredients in a large bowl.

Place in an airtight container until ready to use.

165 Nut Butter Maple Dip

Preparation time: 1 hourCooking time: 1 hour Servings:
Ingredients:

½ tablespoon ground flaxseed1 teaspoon ground cinnamon
½ tablespoon maple syrup

2 tablespoons cashew milk

¾ cups crunchy, unsweetened peanut butterDirections:
In a bowl, combine the flaxseed, cinnamon, maple syrup, cashew milk and peanut butter.

Use a fork to mix everything in. I stir it like I'm scrambling eggs. The mixture should be creamy. If it's too runny, add a little more peanut butter; if it's too thick, add a little more cashew milk.

Refrigerate for about an hour, covered and serve.

Smoothies and Beverages

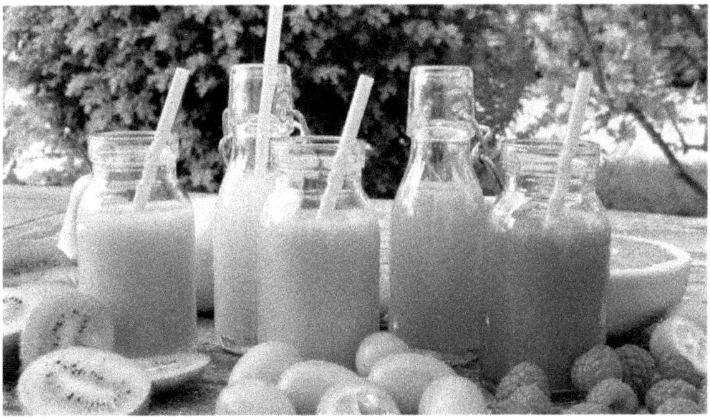

166 Kale & Avocado Smoothie

Preparation Time: 10 MinutesCooking time: 0 minute Servings: 1
Ingredients:

1 ripe banana

1 cup kale

1 cup almond milk

¼ avocado

1 tbsp. chia seeds2 tsp. honey
1 cup ice cubes

Direction:

Blend all the ingredients until smooth.

Nutrition: Calories 343 Total Fat 14 gSaturated Fat 2 g Cholesterol 0 mgSodium 199 mgTotal Carbohydrate 55 g Dietary Fiber 12 g Protein 6 gTotal Sugars 29 gPotassium 1051mg

167 Coconut & Strawberry Smoothie

Preparation Time: 10 MinutesCooking Time: 0 minutes Serves: 1
Calories: 278

Protein: 14 Grams

Fat: 2 Grams

Carbs: 57 GramsIngredients:
1 Cup Strawberries, Frozen & Thawed Slightly

1 Ripe Banana, Sliced & Frozen

½ Cup Coconut Milk, Light

½ Cup Vegan Yogurt

1 Tablespoon Chia Seeds

1 Teaspoon Lime juice, Fresh4 Ice Cubes
Directions:

Blend everything together until smooth, and serve immediately.

168 Pumpkin Chia Smoothie

Preparation Time: 5 MinutesCooking Time: 0 minutes Serves: 1
Calories: 726

Protein: 5.5 Grams

Fat: 69.8 Grams

Carbs: 15 GramsIngredients:
3 Tablespoons Pumpkin Puree

1 Tablespoon MCT Oil

¾ Cup Coconut Milk, Full Fat

½ Avocado, Fresh

1 Teaspoon Vanilla, Pure

½ Teaspoon Pumpkin Pie SpiceDirections:
Combine all ingredients together until blended.

169 Mini Berry Tarts

Preparation Time: 35 minutes + 1 hour chillingServings: 4
Tickle-sized berries-filled with surprises, oh so delicious! Also so delicious that you can't stop having them.

Ingredients

For the piecrust:

4 tbsp flax seed powder + 12 tbsp water

1/3 cup whole-wheat flour + more for dusting

½ tsp salt

¼ cup plant butter, cold and crumbled3 tbsp pure malt syrup
1 ½ tsp vanilla extractFor the filling:
6 oz cashew cream

6 tbsp pure date sugar

¾ tsp vanilla extract

1 cup mixed frozen berriesDirections
Preheat the oven to 350 F and grease a mini pie pans with cooking

spray.

In a medium bowl, mix the flax seed powder with water and allow soaking for 5 minutes.

In a large bowl, combine the flour and salt. Add the butter and usingan electric hand mixer, whisk until crumbly. Pour in the flax egg, malt

syrup, vanilla, and mix until smooth dough forms.

Flatten the dough on a flat surface, cover with plastic wrap, and refrigerate for 1 hour.

After, lightly dust a working surface with some flour, remove the dough onto the surface, and using a rolling pin, flatten the dough into a 1-inch diameter circle,

Use a large cookie cutter, cut out rounds of the dough and fit into thepie pans. Use a knife to trim the edges of the pan. Lay a parchment paper on the dough cups, pour on some baking beans and bake in the oven until golden brown, 15 to 20 minutes.

Remove the pans from the oven, pour out the baking beans, and allow cooling.

In a medium bowl, mix the cashew cream, date sugar, and vanilla extract.

Divide the mixture into the tart cups and top with berries. Serve immediately.

Nutritional info per serving

Calories 545 | Fats 33.5g| Carbs 53.6g | Protein 10.6g

170 Mixed Nut Chocolate Fudge

Preparation Time: 2 hours 10 minutes

Servings: 4

A recipe for chocolate fudge that takes just 10 minutes to make and requires ingredients that are readily available.

Ingredients

3 cups unsweetened chocolate chips

¼ cup thick coconut milk

1 ½ tsp vanilla extractA pinch salt

1 cup chopped mixed nuts

Directions

Line a 9-inch square pan with baking paper and set aside.

Melt the chocolate chips, coconut milk, and vanilla in a medium pot over low heat.

Mix in the salt and nuts until well distributed and pour the mixture into the square pan.

Refrigerate for at least for at least 2 hours.

Remove from the fridge, cut into squares and serve. Nutritional info per serving

Calories 907 | Fats 31.5g| Carbs 152.1g | Protein 7.7g

171 Date Cake Slices

Preparation Time: 1 hour 20 minutes

Servings: 4

With a slightly thick yet fluffy texture, they're super soft.Ingredients
½ cup cold plant butter, cut in pieces, plus extra for greasing1 tbsp flax seed powder + 3 tbsp water
½ cup whole-wheat flour, plus extra for dusting

¼ cup chopped pecans and walnuts1 tsp baking powder
1 tsp baking soda

1 tsp cinnamon powder

3 tsp salt

1/3 cup water

1/3 cup pitted dates, chopped

½ cup pure date sugar1 tsp vanilla extract
¼ cup pure date syrup for drizzling.

Directions

Preheat the oven to 350 F and lightly grease a round baking dish with some plant butter.

In a small bowl, mix the flax seed powder with water and allow thickening for 5 minutes to make the flax egg.

In a food processor, add the flour, nuts, baking powder, baking soda, cinnamon powder, and salt. Blend until well combined.

Add the water, dates, date sugar, and vanilla. Process until smooth with tiny pieces of dates evident.

Pour the batter into the baking dish and bake in the oven for 1 hour and 10 minutes or until a toothpick inserted comes out clean. Remove the dish from the oven, invert the cake onto a servingplatter to cool, drizzle with the date syrup, slice, and serve.

Nutritional info per serving

Calories 850 | Fats 61.2g| Carbs 65.7g | Protein 12.8g

172 Chocolate Mousse Cake

Preparation Time: 40 minutes + 6 hours 30 minutes chillingServings: 4

Have a cake with a basic mousse of chocolate and tell me how youfeel.

Ingredients

2/3 cup toasted almond flour

¼ cup unsalted plant butter, melted

4 cups unsweetened chocolate bars, broken into pieces2 ½ cups coconut cream

Fresh raspberries or strawberries for toppingDirections

Lightly grease a 9-inch springform pan with some plant butter andset aside.

Mix the almond flour and plant butter in a medium bowl and pour the mixture into the springform pan. Use the spoon to spread and press the mixture into the bottom of the pan. Place in the refrigerator tofirm for 30 minutes.

Meanwhile, pour the chocolate in a safe microwave bowl and meltfor 1 minute stirring every 30 seconds.

Remove from the microwave and mix in the coconut cream and maple syrup.

Remove the cake pan from the oven, pour the chocolate mixture on top making to sure to shake the pan and even the layer. Chill further for 4 to 6 hours.

Take out the pan from the fridge, release the cake and garnish with the raspberries or strawberries.

Slice and serve. Nutritional info per serving

Calories 608 | Fats 60.5g| Carbs 19.8g | Protein 6.3g

Snacks and Desserts

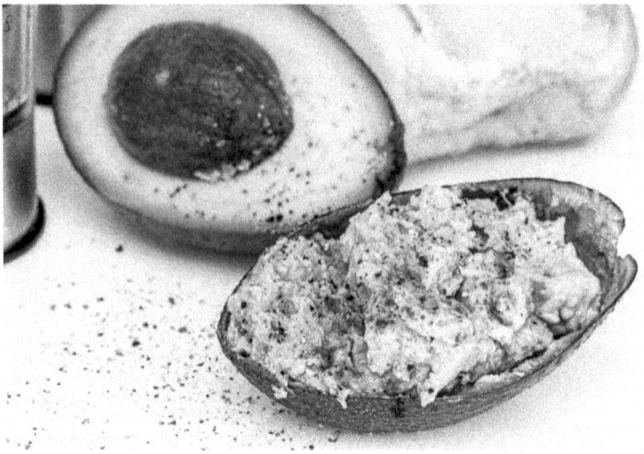

173 Nori Snack Rolls

Preparation Time: 5 minutesCooking time: 10 minutes Servings: 4 rolls
Ingredients

2 tablespoons almond, cashew, peanut, or others nut butter2 tablespoons tamari, or soy sauce
4 standard nori sheets

1 mushroom, sliced

1 tablespoon pickled ginger

½ cup grated carrotsDirections
Preparing the Ingredients. Preheat the oven to 350°F.
Mix together the nut butter and tamari until smooth and very thick. Lay out a nori sheet, rough side up, the long way.

Spread a thin line of the tamari mixture on the far end of the nori sheet, from side to side. Lay the mushroom slices, ginger, andcarrots in a line at the other end (the end closest to you).

Fold the vegetables inside the nori, rolling toward the tahini mixture, which will seal the roll. Repeat to make 4 rolls.

Put on a baking sheet and bake for 8 to 10 minutes, or until the rolls are slightly browned and crispy at the ends. Let the rolls cool for a few minutes, then slice each roll into 3 smaller pieces.

Nutrition: Calories: 79; Total fat: 5g; Carbs: 6g; Fiber: 2g; Protein: 4g

174 Risotto Bites

Preparation Time: 15 minutesCooking time: 20 minutes Servings: 12 bites
Ingredients

½ cup panko bread crumbs1 teaspoon paprika

3 teaspoon chipotle powder or ground cayenne pepper

1½ cups cold Green Pea RisottoNonstick cooking spray Directions
Preparing the Ingredients. Preheat the oven to 425°F.
Line a baking sheet with parchment paper.

On a large plate, combine the panko, paprika, and chipotle powder. Set aside.

Roll 2 tablespoons of the risotto into a ball.

Gently roll in the bread crumbs, and place on the prepared baking sheet. Repeat to make a total of 12 balls.

Spritz the tops of the risotto bites with nonstick cooking spray and bake for 15 to 20 minutes, until they begin to brown. Cool completely before storing in a large airtight container in a single layer (add a piece of parchment paper for a second layer) or in a plastic freezer bag.

Nutrition: Calories: 100; Fat: 2g; Protein: 6g; Carbohydrates: 17g; Fiber: 5g; Sugar: 2g; Sodium: 165 mg

175 Jicama and Guacamole

Preparation Time: 15 minutesCooking time: 0 minutes Servings: 4
Ingredients

juice of 1 lime, or 1 tablespoon prepared lime juice

4 hass avocados, peeled, pits removed, and cut into cubes

½ teaspoon sea salt

½ red onion, minced 1 garlic clove, minced
¼ cup chopped cilantro (optional)

1 jicama bulb, peeled and cut into matchsticksDirections
Preparing the Ingredients.

In a medium bowl, squeeze the lime juice over the top of theavocado and sprinkle with salt.

Lightly mash the avocado with a fork. Stir in the onion, garlic, and cilantro, if using.

Serve with slices of jicama to dip in guacamole.

To store, place plastic wrap over the bowl of guacamole and refrigerate. The guacamole will keep for about 2 days.

176 Oven-baked Caramelize Plantains

Preparation time: 30 minutesCooking time: 17 minutes Servings: 4
Ingredients

4 medium plantains, peeled and sliced2 Tbsp fresh orange juice
4 Tbsp brown sugar or to taste

1 Tbsp grated orange zest

4 Tbsp coconut butter, meltedDirections
Preheat oven to 360 F/180 C.

Place plantain slices in a heatproof dish.

Pour the orange juice over plantains, and then sprinkle with brown sugar and grated orange zest.

Melt coconut butter and pour evenly over plantains. Cover with foil and bake for 15 to 17 minutes.
Serve warm or cold with honey or maple syrup.

177 Powerful Peas & Lentils Dip

Preparation time: 10 minutesCooking time: 0 minutes Servings: 4
Ingredients

4 cups frozen peas

2 cup green lentils cooked1 piece of grated ginger
1/2 cup fresh basil chopped1 cup ground almonds Juice of 1/2 lime
Pinch of salt

4 Tbsp sesame oil

1/4 cup Sesame seedsDirections
Place all ingredients in a food processor or in a blender.

Blend until all ingredients combined well.

Keep refrigerated in an airtight container up to 4 days.

178 Protein "Raffaello" Candies

Preparation time: 15 minutesCooking time: 0 minutes Servings: 12
Ingredients

1 1/2 cups desiccated coconut flakes1/2 cup coconut butter softened
4 Tbsp coconut milk canned

4 Tbs coconut palm sugar (or granulated sugar) 1 tsp pure vanilla extract1 Tbsp vegan protein powder (pea or soy)15 whole almonds
Directions

Put 1 cup of desiccated coconut flakes, and all remaining ingredientsin the blender (except almonds), and blend until soft.

If your dough is too thick, add some coconut milk. In a bowl, add remaining coconut flakes.
Coat every almond in one tablespoon of mixture and roll into a ball. Roll each ball in coconut flakes.
Chill in the fridge for several hours.

179 Roasted Cauliflower

Preparation Time: 30 MinutesCooking Time: 20 Minutes Servings: 4
Ingredients:

Olive Oil (1 T.) Cauliflower (1, Chopped)Salt (to Taste)

Smoked Paprika (2 t.)Parsley (2 T.) Directions:

If you like to snack, it is better to have healthier options at hand. You'll want to start this recipe off by prepping your oven to 450.

As this warms up, place the cauliflower florets into a large mixing bowl and toss with the olive oil, salt, and smoked paprika. Once this is complete, lay it across a baking sheet and pop it into the oven for 20 minutes.

When the cauliflower is cooked to your liking, remove from the oven, top with parsley, and you are all set.

Nutrition: Calories: 70 Proteins: 3g Carbs: 8g Fats: 5g

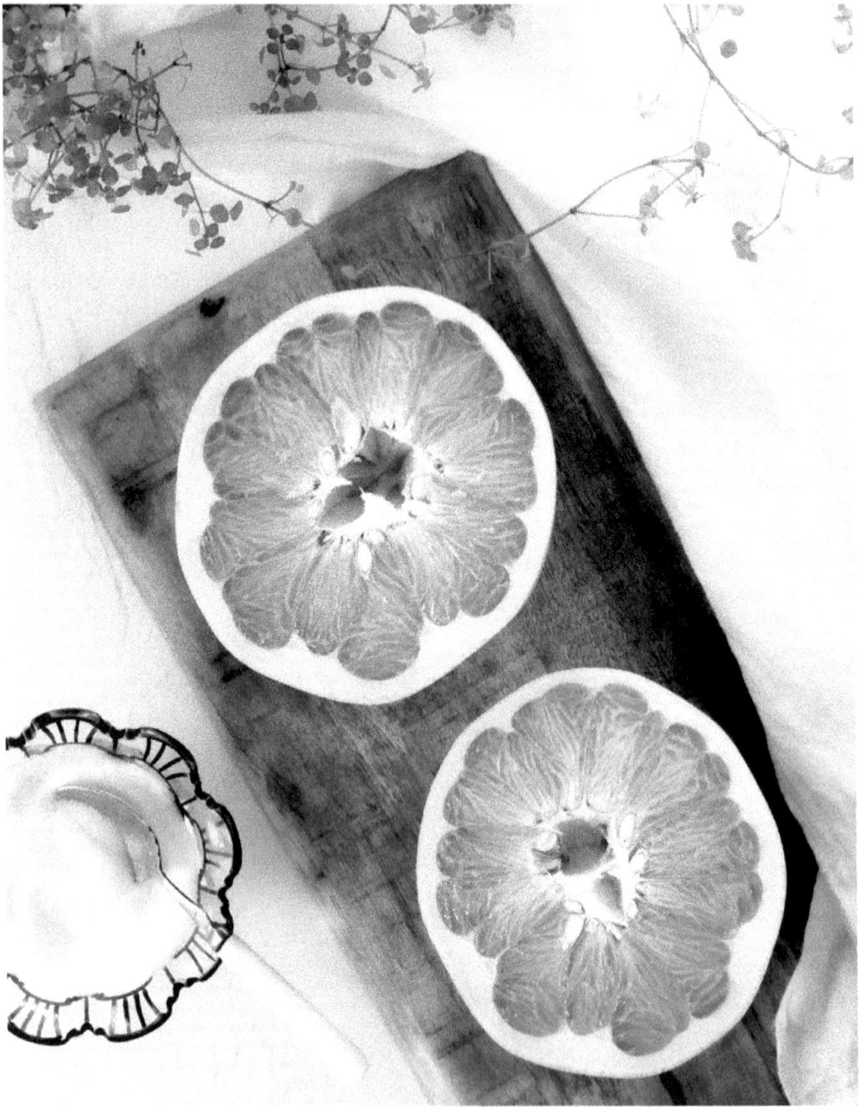

Dinner Recipes

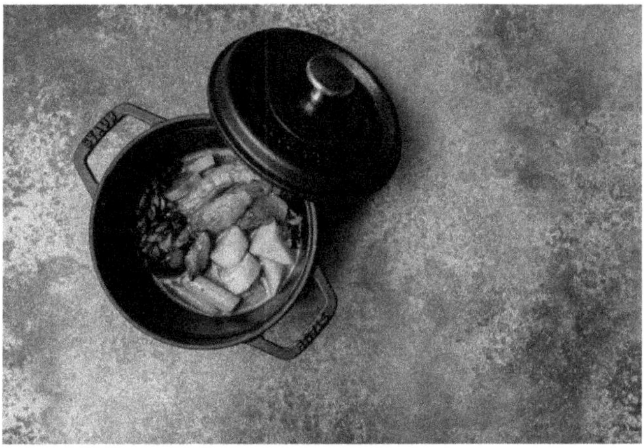

180 Cauliflower Steak Kicking Corn

Preparation: 30 min.Cooking: 60 min.Servings: 6

Ingredients:

2 t. capers, drained 4 scallions, chopped1 red chili, minced
¼ c. vegetable oil

2 ears of corn, shucked 2 big cauliflower heads Salt and pepper to taste
Directions:
Heat the oven to 375 degrees.

Boil a pot of water, about 4 cups, using the maximum heat setting available.

Add corn in the saucepan, cooking approximately 3 minutes or until tender.

Drain and allow the corn to cool, then slice the kernels away from thecob.

Warm 2 tablespoons of vegetable oil in a skillet.

Combine the chili pepper with the oil, cooking for approximately 30 seconds.

Next, combine the scallions, sautéing with the chili pepper until soft. Mix in the corn and capers in the skillet and cook for approximately 1 minute to blend the flavors. Then remove from heat. Warm 1 tablespoon of vegetable oil in a skillet. Once warm, begin to place cauliflower steaks to the pan, 2 to 3 at a time. Season to your liking with salt and cook over medium heat for 3 minutes or until lightly browned. Once cooked, slide onto the cookie sheet and repeat step 5 with the remaining cauliflower.

Take the corn mixture and press into the spaces between the florets of the cauliflower.

Bake for 25 minutes. Serve warm and enjoy!
Nutrition: Calories: 153 | Carbohydrates: 15 g | Proteins: 4 g | Fats:10 g

181 Green beans stir fry

Preparation time 30 minutes

Cooking time: 10 minutesServings: 6-8 Ingredients:

1 1/2 pounds of green beans, stringed, chopped into 1 ½-inchpieces

1 large onion, thinly sliced4 star anise (optional)

3 tablespoons avocado oil

3 1/2 tablespoons tamari sauce or soy sauceSalt to taste

3/4 cup water

Direction:

Place a wok over medium heat. Add oil. When oil is heated, add onions and sauté until onions are translucent.

Add beans, water, tamari sauce, and star anise and stir. Cover andcook until the beans are tender.

Uncover, add salt and raise the heat to high. Cook until the water dries up in the wok. Stir a couple of times while cooking.

182 Mean bean minestrone

Preparation time: 45 minutesCooking time: 40 minutes Servings: 6
Protein content per serving: 9gIngredients
1 tablespoon (15 ml) olive oil

1/3 cup (80 g) chopped red onion

4 cloves garlic, grated or pressed

3 leek, white and light green parts, trimmed and chopped (about 4 ounces, or 113 g)

4 carrots, peeled and minced (about 4 ounces, or 113 g)2 ribs of celery, minced (about 2 ounces, or 57 g)
2 yellow squashes, trimmed and chopped (about 8 ounces, or 227 g) 1 green bell pepper, trimmed and chopped (about 8 ounces, or 227 g)
1 tablespoon (16 g) tomato paste1 teaspoon dried oregano
4 teaspoon dried basil

⅓ teaspoon smoked paprika

'¼ To ¼ teaspoon cayenne pepper, or to taste

5 cans (each 15 ounces, or 425 g) diced fire-roasted tomatoes4 cups (940 ml) vegetable broth, more if needed

6 cups (532 g) cannellini beans, or other white beans

2 cups (330 g) cooked farro, or other whole grain or pastaSalt, to taste
Nut and seed sprinkles, for garnish, optional and to tasteDirections:
In a large pot, add the oil, onion, garlic, leek, carrots, celery, yellow

squash, bell pepper, tomato paste, oregano, basil, paprika, and cayenne pepper. Cook on medium-high heat, stirring often until the vegetables start to get tender, about 6 minutes.

Add the tomatoes and broth. Bring to a boil, lower the heat, cover with a lid, and simmer 15 minutes.

Add the beans and simmer another 10 minutes. Add the farro and simmer 5 more minutes to heat the farro.

Note that this is a thick minestrone. If there are leftovers (which tasteeven better, by the way), the soup will thicken more once chilled.

Add extra broth if you prefer a thinner soup and adjust seasoning if needed. Add nut and seed sprinkles on each portion upon serving, if desired.

Store leftovers in an airtight container in the refrigerator for up to 5 days. The minestrone can also be frozen for up to 3 months.

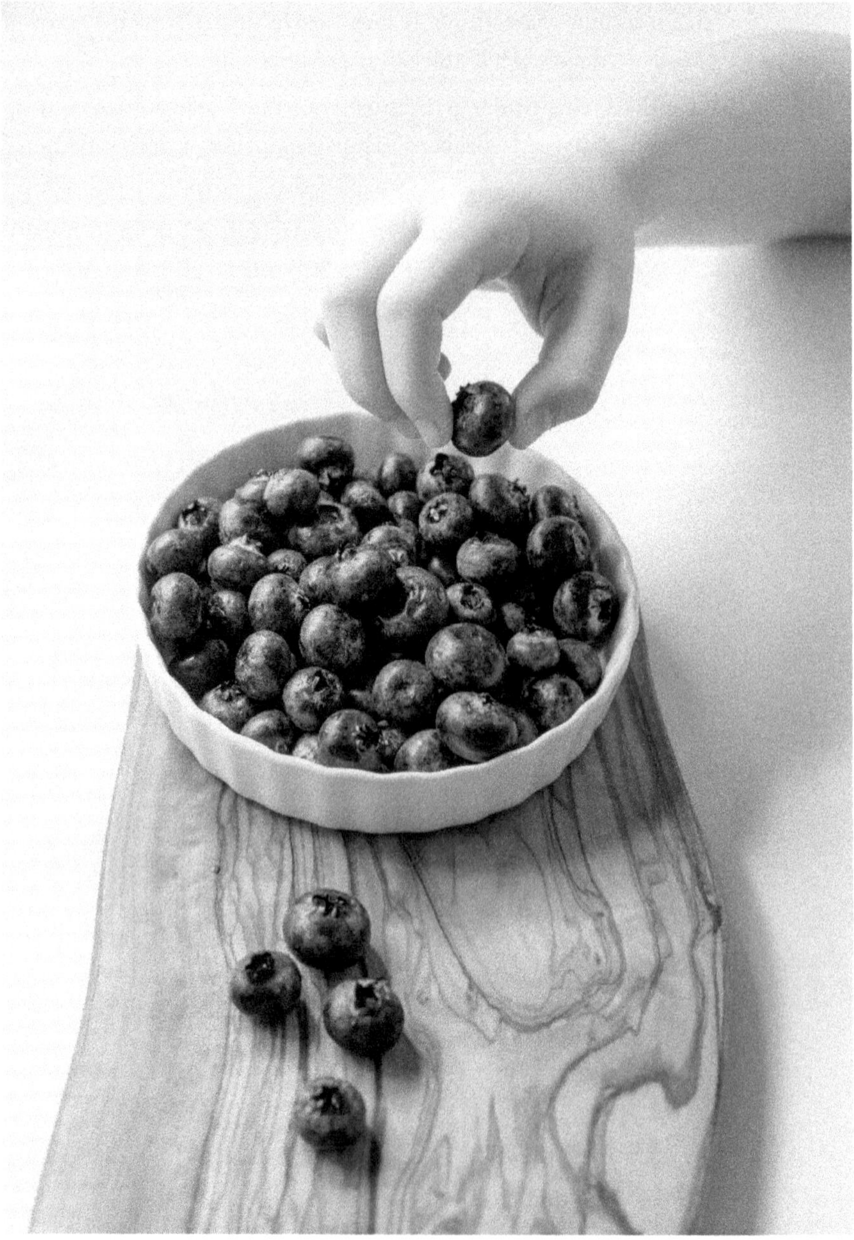

Lunch Recipes

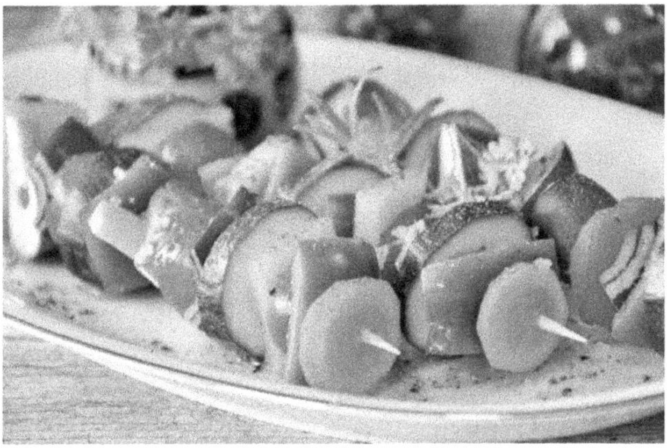

183 Chickpea And Edamame Salad

Preparation Time: 40 minutesCooking Time: 0 minutes Serving: 4
Ingredients:

For the Salad:

4 tablespoons dried cranberries 1/4 cup (59 grams) diced carrots
3/4 cup (177 grams) edamame soybeans 1/3 cup (78 grams) chopped green pepper30 ounces (850 grams) cooked chickpeas1/3 cup (78 grams) chopped red pepper 1/2 teaspoon minced garlic
For the Dressing:

1/4 teaspoon dried oregano1 teaspoon coconut sugar 1/4 teaspoon dried basil
1/3 teaspoon ground black pepper

1/3 teaspoon salt

1/4 teaspoon dried rosemary1 teaspoon white vinegar
2 tablespoons grape seed oil2 tablespoons olive oil Directions:
Preparethe salad: takealargesaladbowl, place allsalad ingredients in it and then toss until properly mixed.

Preparehe dressing:takeasmall bowl,placealldressingingredients in it and then whisk until combined.

Drizzle dressing over salad and toss until well mixed.

Place the salad bowl in the refrigerator for at least 30 minutes until chilled, then serve.

Nutrition: 119.6 Cal; 1.9 g Fat; 0.1 g Saturated Fat; 20.8 g Carbs; 4.8 g Fiber; 6 g Protein; 1.1 g Sugar;

184 Cauliflower Salad

Preparation Time: 20 minutesCooking Time: 15 minutes Servings: 4
Ingredients:

8 cups cauliflower florets

5 tablespoons olive oil, dividedSalt and pepper to taste
1 cup parsley

3 clove garlic, minced

4 tablespoons lemon juice

¼ cup almonds, toasted and sliced3 cups arugula
2 tablespoons olives, sliced

¼ cup feta, crumbledDirection
Preheat your oven to 425 degrees F.

Toss the cauliflower in a mixture of 1 tablespoon olive oil, salt and pepper.Place in a baking pan and roast for 15 minutes.Put the parsley, remaining oil, garlic, lemon juice, salt and pepper ina blender.Pulse until smooth.

Place the roasted cauliflower in a salad bowl.

Stir in the rest of the ingredients along with the parsley dressing.

Nutrition: Calories: 198 Total fat: 16.5g Saturated fat: 3g Cholesterol:6mg Sodium: 3mg Potassium: 570mg Carbohydrates: 10.4g Fiber: 4.1g Sugar: 4g Protein: 5.4g

185 Garlic Mashed Potatoes & Turnips

Preparation: 20 minutesCooking: 30 minutes Servings: 8
Ingredients:

1 head garlic 1 teaspoon olive oil lb. turnips, sliced into cubes lb. potatoes, sliced into cubes

½ cup almond milk

½ cup vegan parmesan cheese, grated1 tablespoon fresh thyme, chopped

3 tablespoon fresh chives, chopped2 tablespoons vegan butter
Salt and pepper to tasteDirection
Preheat your oven to 375 degrees F.Slice the tip off the garlic head.
Drizzle with a little oil and roast in the oven for 45 minutes.

Boil the turnips and potatoes in a pot of water for 30 minutes or until tender.

Add all the ingredients to a food processor along with the garlic. Pulse until smooth.

Nutrition: Calories: 141 Total fat: 3.2g Saturated fat: 1.5g Cholesterol: 7mg Sodium: 284mg Potassium: 676mgCarbohydrates: 24.6g Fiber: 3.1g Sugar: 4g Protein: 4.6g

186 Pulled "Pork" Sandwiches

This pulled "pork" is the perfect dish to make ahead. Prepare the mushrooms and coat them in the sauce and then you can store them chilled in the cold-storage box or the icebox. If you prepare a large amount to keep in the icebox, you will always have some on hand for sandwiches, pizza, nachos, or any other vegan-version of popular dishes that might be complemented by pulled "pork".

Preparation time: 40 minutesCooking Time: 35 minutes Servings: 3
Ingredients:

King oyster mushrooms* – 4 Barbecue sauce – .25 cup Olive oil – 2 tablespoons Sea salt – .25 teaspoon Garlic, minced – 2 cloves
Cayenne pepper – .25 teaspoonBread – 6 slices
Directions:

Start by setting your electric cooker to Fahrenheit 400 degrees.

While your electric cooker warms up, clean the mushrooms with a damp paper towel and then use two forks to shred both the caps and stems of the mushrooms into pieces resembling pulled pork. Place

the shredded mushrooms on a kitchen parchment-lined aluminum baking sheet.

Drizzle the mushrooms with half of the olive oil and then toss them with the seasoning and garlic until evenly coated. Allow the oyster mushrooms to roast until slightly crispy and browned about twenty minutes.

In a skillet, add the remaining tablespoon of olive oil, allowing it to warm over midway-elevated. Put the cooked mushrooms in the pan along with the barbecue sauce.

Cook the mushrooms in the sauce while stirring until the sauce is fragrant and warm, about three to five minutes. Top three slices of bread with this concoction and top with the remaining three slices. Cut the sandwiches in half before serving. Note:

*If you can't find king oyster mushrooms, then you can use three heaping cups of regular oyster mushrooms.

Nutrition: Calories 259

187 Coconut zucchini cream

Preparation time: 10 minutesCooking time: 25 minutes Servings: 4
Ingredients:

1 pound zucchinis, roughly chopped2 tablespoons avocado oil
4 scallions, chopped

Salt and black pepper to the taste6 cups veggie stock
1 teaspoon basil, dried

1 teaspoon cumin, ground3 garlic cloves, minced
¾ cup coconut cream

1 tablespoon dill, choppedDirections:
Heat up a pot with the oil over medium high heat, add the scallions and the garlic and sauté for 5 minutes.

Add the rest of the ingredients, stir, bring to a simmer and cook over medium heat for 20 minutes more.

Blend the soup using an immersion blender, ladle into bowls and serve.

Nutrition: calories 160, fat 4, fiber 2, carbs 4, protein 8

188 Zucchini and Cauliflower Soup

Preparation time: 10 minutesCooking time: 25 minutes

Servings: 4Ingredients:
4 scallions, chopped

1 teaspoon ginger, grated2 tablespoons olive oil

3 pound zucchinis, sliced

4 cups cauliflower florets

Salt and black pepper to the taste6 cups veggie stock
1 garlic clove, minced

1 tablespoon lemon juice1 cup coconut cream Directions:
Heat up a pot with the oil over medium heat, add the scallions, ginger and the garlic and sauté for 5 minutes.

Add the rest of the ingredients, bring to a simmer and cook over medium heat for 20 minutes.

Blend everything using an immersion blender, ladle into soup bowlsand serve.

Nutrition: calories 154, fat 12, fiber 3, carbs 5, protein 4

189 Chard soup

Preparation time: 10 minutesCooking time: 25 minutes Servings: 4
Ingredients:

1 pound Swiss chard, chopped

½ cup shallots, chopped 1 tablespoon avocado oil 1 teaspoon cumin, ground

3 teaspoon rosemary, dried1 teaspoon basil, dried

4 garlic cloves, minced

Salt and black pepper to the taste6 cups vegetable stock
1 tablespoon tomato passata

1 tablespoon cilantro, choppedDirections:
Heat up a pan with the oil over medium heat, add the shallots and the garlic and sauté for 5 minutes.

Add the swiss chard and the other ingredients, toss, bring to asimmer and cook over medium heat for 20 minutes more.

Divide the soup into bowls and serve.

Nutrition: calories 232, fat 23, fiber 3, carbs 4, protein 3

190 Eggplant and Olives Stew

Preparation time: 10 minutesCooking time: 30 minutes Servings: 4
Ingredients:

3 scallions, chopped

2 tablespoons avocado oil

2 garlic cloves, chopped 1 bunch parsley, chopped
Salt and black pepper to the taste

3 teaspoon basil, dried 1 teaspoon cumin, dried
4 eggplants, roughly cubed

1 cup green olives, pitted and sliced3 tablespoons balsamic vinegar
½ Cup tomato passataDirections:
Heat up a pot with the oil over medium heat, add the scallions, garlic,basil and cumin and sauté for 5 minutes.

Add the eggplants and the other ingredients, toss, cook over mediumheat for 25 minutes more, divide into bowls and serve.

Nutrition: calories 93, fat 1.8, fiber 10.6, carbs 18.6, protein 3.4

Recipes For Main Courses And Single Dishes

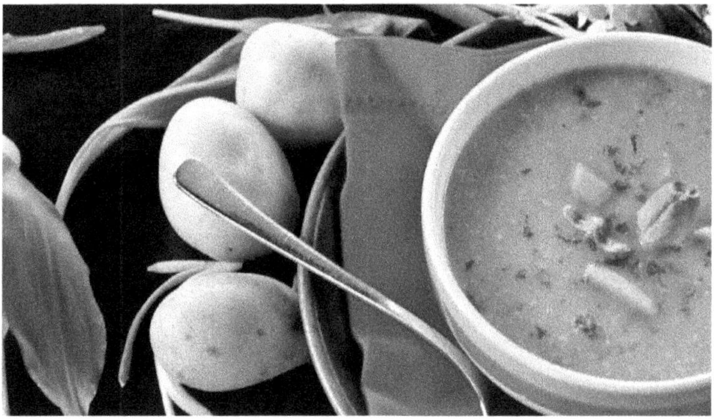

191 Pecan & Blueberry Crumble

Preparation Time: 40 MinutesCooking Time: 1 Hour Servings: 6
Calories: 381

Protein: 10 Grams

Fat: 32 Grams

Net Carbs: 20 GramsIngredients:
14 Ounces Blueberries

1 Tablespoon Lemon Juice, Fresh1 ½ Teaspoon Stevia Powder
3 Tablespoons Chia Seeds

2 Cups Almond Flour, Blanched

¼ Cup Pecans, Chopped 5 Tablespoon coconut Oil 2 Tablespoon Cinnamon Directions:
Mix together your blueberries, stevia, chia seeds and lemon juice,and place it in an iron skillet.

Mix ingredients while spreading it over your blueberries.

Heat your oven to 400, and then transfer it to an oven safe skillet, baking for a half hour.

Interesting Facts: Blueberries: These guys are a delectable treat thatis easily incorporated into many dishes. They are packed with antioxidants and Vitamin C. Bonus: Blueberries have been proven to promote eye health and slow macular degeneration.

192 Rice Pudding

Preparation Time: 1 Hour 35 Minutes Cooking Time: 1 Hour and 30 MinutesServings: 6
Ingredients:

1 Cup Brown Rice

1 Teaspoon Vanilla Extract, Pure

½ Teaspoon Sea Salt, Fine

½ Teaspoon Cinnamon

¼ Teaspoon Nutmeg3 Egg Substitutes
3 Cups Coconut Milk, Light

2 Cups Brown Rice, CookedDirections:
Blend all of your ingredients together before pouring them into a two quarter dish.

Bake at 300 for ninety minutes before serving.

Interesting Facts: Brown rice is incredibly high in antioxidants and good vitamins. It's relative, 14 white rice is far less beneficial asmuch of these healthy nutrients get destroyed during the process of milling. You can also opt for red and black rice or wild rice. The meal options for this healthy grain are limitless!

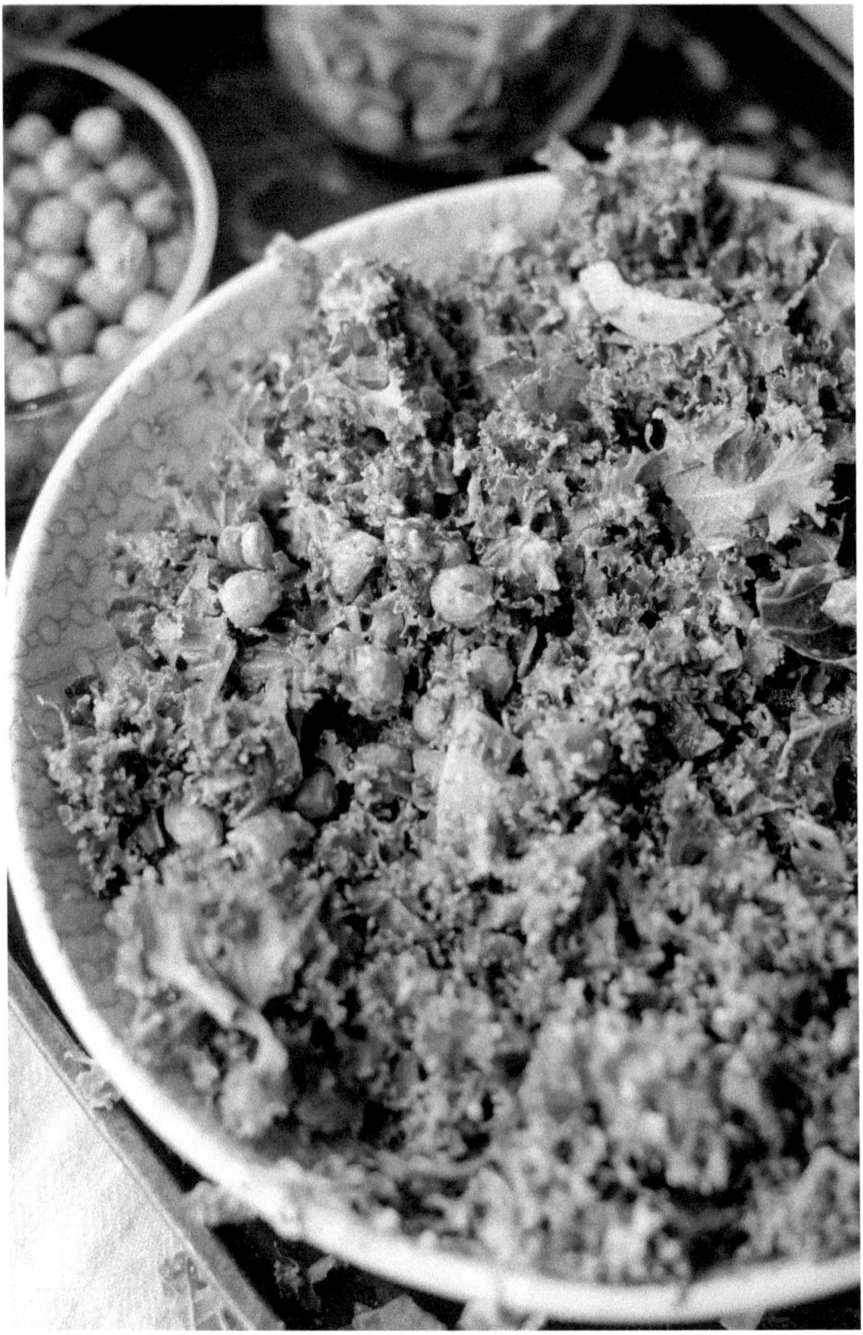

Nutrient-Packed Protein Salads

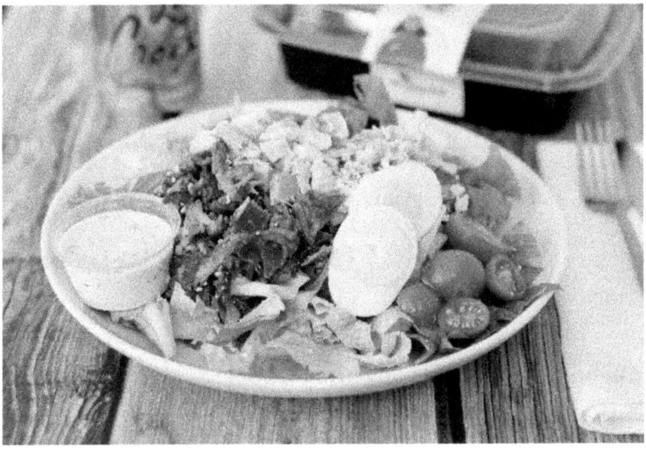

193 Chickpea, Red Kidney Bean And Feta Salad

Preparation time: 5 minsCooking time: 5 mins Ingredient:

1 can chickpeas

1 can red kidney beans

1 piece small of ginger grated or shredded1 medium onion diced
2- 3 cloves garlic

1 tbsp olive oil

A pinch of red chili flakes

3-4 spring onions green part only, chopped, scallions 1 cup chopped parsley OR coriander I used cilantro Juice of one lemon150 g feta cheese – almost half cup sizeSalt and Black pepper.

Directions:

Heat 1 tablespoon of olive oil and cook the onion till lightly golden. Do not overdo it and the onions should still be crunchy. Add garlic, ginger and chili and cook till the garlic is fragrant. Set aside to cool so it doesn't melt the feta when you mix it in. Drain the chickpeasand red kidney beans, rinse and place in the salad bowl. Add crumbled feta, spring onion, parsley (or coriander) and lemon juice, season with salt and pepper. Add the cooled onion and garlic mixtureand remaining oil and mix well.

194 Curried Carrot Slaw With Tempeh

Preparation: 10 minsCooking: 10 mins

Ingredient:

8 ounces tempeh, sliced into triangles 1/4 tsp liquid smoke (optional) 1 1/2 Tbsp maple syrup, grade B

1 tsp extra virgin olive oil or virgin coconut oil 2-3 tsp tamari or 2 tsp soy sauce

1 Tbsp crushed raw walnuts4 cups shredded carrots

1 small onion, diced 1 Tbsp curry powder

1/4 tsp turmeric powder (for added turmeric power, optional) 1/8 tsp black pepper2 Tbsp tahini

1/4 cup fresh lemon juice sweet stuff: 1 – 1 1/2 Tbsp maple syrup + an optional handful orraisins

1/2 cup flat leaf parsley, finely chopped + some for garnish

a few pinches of cayenne for heat (optional)salt and pepper for carrot salad – to taste.

Directions:

Warm a skillet up over high heat and add in the coconut or olive oil. When oil is hot, add the tempeh triangles, tamari, maple and liquid smoke. Flip the tempeh around a bit to allow it to absorb the liquid. Cook for about 5 minutes, flipping the tempeh a few times throughout the cooking process. When tempeh is browned and edges blackened a bit, and all liquid absorbed, turn off heat. Sprinkle the walnut pieces and some black pepper over top the tempeh and set pan aside to keep triangles warm in skillet. In a large mixing bowl, add the carrots, tahini, lemon juice, spices, parsley, maple syrup, optional raisins and onion. Toss very well for a few minutes to marinate the carrots with the dressing. For a creamier salad, add another spoonful of tahini. To thin things out and make the salad zestier, add another splash of lemon juice or a teaspoon of apple cider vinegar. Finally, add salt and pepper to the carrot salad to taste. Pour the carrot salad in a large serving bowl and top with the tempeh. Serve right away or place in the fridge to serve in a few hours or up to a day later. The carrots will soften the longer they set in the fridge.

195 Black & White Bean Quinoa Salad

Preparation time: 15 minsCooking time: 15 mins Ingredient:

⅓ cup (75 mL) quinoa

1 can (19 oz/540 mL) black beans, drained and rinsed

1 can (19 oz/540 mL) navy beans, drained and rinsed1 cup (250 mL) diced cucumbers

¼ cup (50 mL) diced red onion

3 jalapeno pepper, seeded and minced (I've never used it and findthe dish spicy enough for me, but feel free to add it if you like things hot!)

¼ cup (50 mL) chopped fresh coriander (cilantro)

¼ cup (50 mL) vegetable oil (I use cold pressed extra-virgin olive oil)

4 tbsp (25 mL) lime juice

1 tbsp (15 mL) cider vinegar1 clove garlic, minced

½ tsp (2 mL) chili powder

1 tsp (5 mL) ground coriander

½ tsp (2 mL) dried oregano

¼ tsp (1 mL) salt

¼ tsp (1 mL) pepper.

Directions:

In saucepan of boiling salted ⅔ C water, cook quinoa until tender, about 12 minutes. Drain and rinse. Dressing: In large bowl, whisk together oil, lime juice, vinegar, garlic, chili powder, coriander, oregano, salt and pepper. Add quinoa, black beans, navy beans, cucumber, onion, jalapeño pepper and coriander; toss to combine.

196 Greek Salad With Seitan Gyros Strips

Preparation time: 5 mins

Cooking time: 5 minsIngredient: 4 tomatoes
1 punnet cherry tomatoes

1 1/2 crunchy cucumbers

3 big handful kalamata olives 1/2 Spanish onion finely sliced
1/4 stick of Cheesy mozzarella style cheese.Fresh oregano and mint
1/4 cup good quality extra virgin olive oil

4 Tablespoons vinegar (red wine or balsamic)1 teaspoon castor sugar
2 teaspoons mixed dried Italian herbs1 clove finely chopped garlic

3 teaspoon soy saucesalt
pepper.

Directions:

In a small frying pan, place gyros strips and fry until slightly blackened on the edges. Leave to cool. Cut up all your veggies roughly and place in a large bowl. Add olives, oregano, mint and chopped cheese. In a jar add all dressing ingredients. Shake welland taste. Combine the cooled gyros strips, salad and dressing and coat well.

197 Chickpea And Edamame Salad

Preparation time: 30 mins

Cooking time: 30 mins

Ingredient: 2 15.5oz each cans chickpea (garbanzo beans) rinsedand drained

3/4 cup edamame soy beans 1/3 cup chopped red pepper 1/3 cup chopped green pepper1/4 cup diced carrots
3 tablespoons dried cranberries1 garlic clove minced
Dressing

2 tablespoons grapeseed oil2 tablespoons olive oil
1 teaspoon white distilled vinegar1 teaspoon sugar
1/4 teaspoon dried oregano1/4 teaspoon dried basil
1/4 teaspoon dried rosemary

Salt and pepperDirections:
In a large bowl combine chickpeas, edamame, red pepper, green

pepper, carrots, dried cranberries, minced garlic and set aside. In a small bowl combine grapeseed oil, olive oil, vinegar, sugar, oregano, basil and rosemary. Whisk until blended. Pour dressing over chick peas and gently toss. Season with salt and pepper to taste. Chill for at least 30 minutes for flavors to blend. Serve chilled.

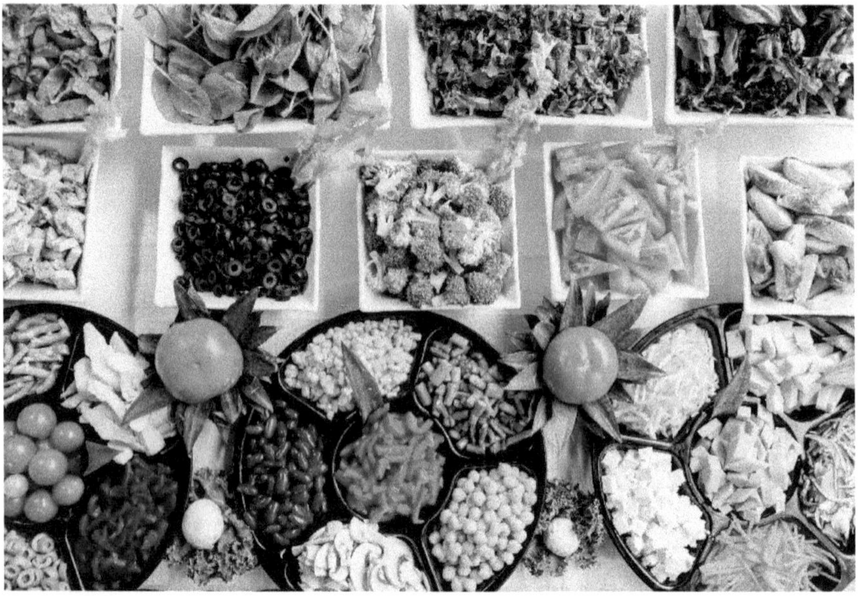

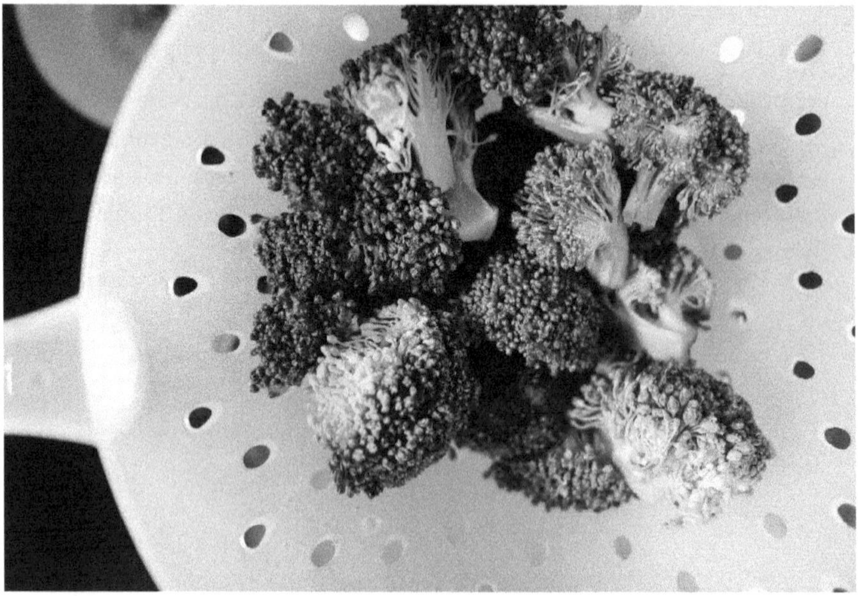

Flavour Boosters (Fish Glazes, Meat Rubs & Fish Rubs)

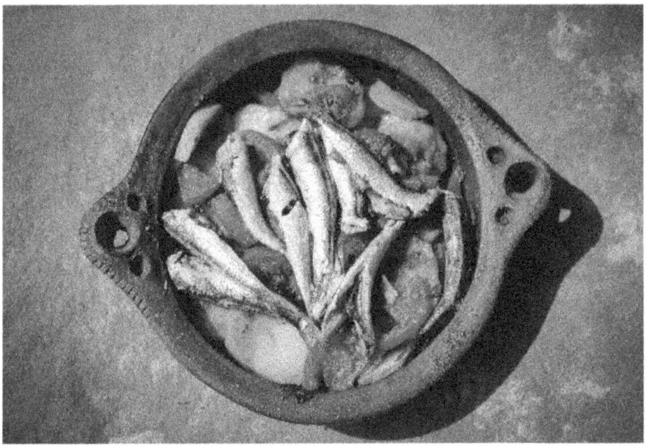

198 Mexican Cocoa Rub

Want to spice up your dry meats with savory Mexican flavors? Tryout my classy rub this weekend. Cocoa and espresso powder are a special addition to this Mexican style rub creating soothing spiced aroma.

Preparation Time: 5 min.Cooking Time: 5 min.
Servings: 9 tsp.

Ingredients:

Water – 1 tbs.

Cocoa, unsweetened – 1 tsp. Instant espresso powder – 2 tsp. Smoked paprika – 2 tsp.
Olive oil – 1 tsp. Ground cumin – 1 tsp.Salt – ¼ tsp.
Directions:

One by one, mix in all the ingredients in your mixing bowl to make the cocoa rub. Gently mix all the ingredients using spatula or spoon to form an aromatic rub mixture.

Now, take your choice of meat cut and place it on a firm surface. Brush or rub the freshly made rub on it; pat gently for the rub to stick to the surface. Turn the meat cut and repeat to spice up its other side. Repeat with other meat cuts.

Let your meat cuts adequately season for more rich flavors for a few hours in your refrigerator. Take them out, as they are ready to be cooked or grilled!

199 Juniper Sage Meat Rub

This unique meat rub has been crafted with quality by including numerous healthy herbs such as juniper berries, lay leaf, red pepper, etc. It delivers piney accent to the rub, which ultimately enhances the flavor of your favorite meat cuts.

Preparation Time: 5 min.Cooking Time: 5 min.
Servings: 8 tsp. Ingredients:

Bay leaf – 1 Black peppercorns - 1 tsp.Juniper berries - 2 tsp. Extra-virgin olive oil - 2 tbs. Crushed red pepper - ½ tsp.Kosher salt - ½ tsp.
Minced garlic – 1 cloveMinced sage leaves - 6Directions:
Mix in the bay leaf, red pepper, salt, peppercorns, and berries in yourspice blender, grinder or processor to make the juniper rub. Start processing or grinding the mixed spiced on "pulse" mode to ground.

Empty the mixed spice mixture in a bowl; mix in the sage leaves, oil, and garlic. Mix again well.

Now, take your choice of meat cut and place it on a firm surface. Brush or rub the freshly made rub on it; pat gently for the rub to stick to the surface. Turn the meat cut and repeat to spice up its other side. Repeat with other meat cuts.

The freshly rubbed meat is ready to be grilled or cooked!

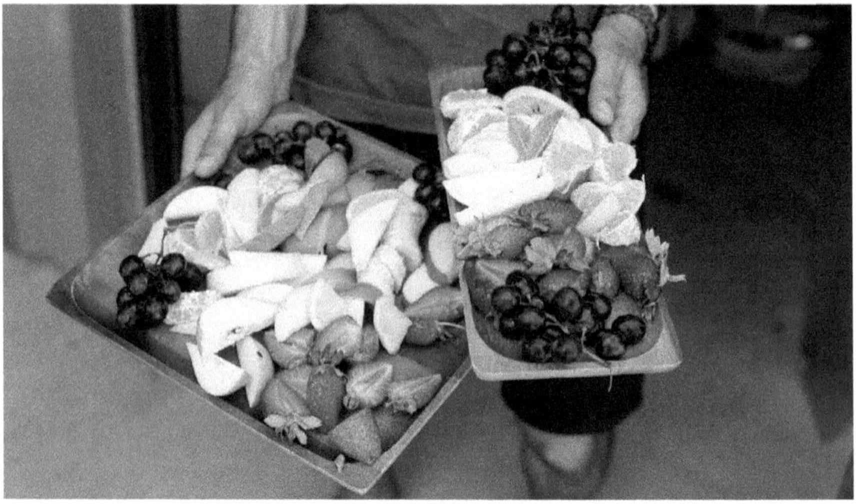

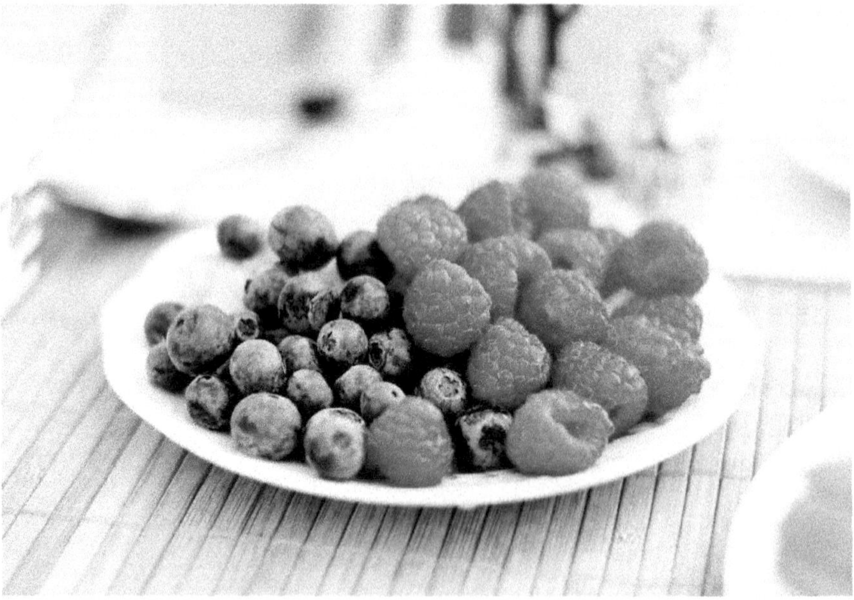

Sauce Recipes

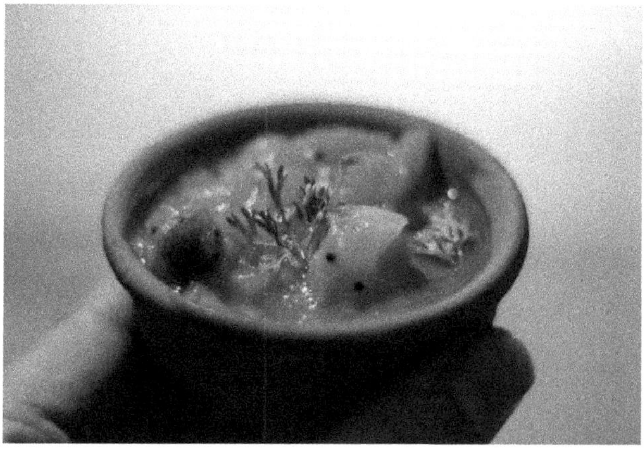

200 Coconut Sugar Peanut Sauce

Preparation time: 5 minutes Cooking time: 5 minute Servings: 1 ½ cups

Ingredients

4 tablespoons coconut sugar

6 tablespoons powdered peanut butter1 tablespoon chili sauce

2 tablespoons liquid aminos

¼ cup of water

1 teaspoon lime juice

½ teaspoon ginger powderDirections:

In a bowl, combine all the ingredients until properly combined. Serve as a topping for the salad or other dishes.Store in a fridge.

Lightning Source UK Ltd.
Milton Keynes UK
UKHW021946140621
385519UK00002B/522

9 781802 896985